G Austin Gresham

A colour atlas of
General
Pathology

G. AUSTIN GRESHAM

T.D., M.D., Sc.D., M.A., M.R.C. Path.

Fellow of Jesus College, Cambridge
Cambridge University Morbid Anatomist and Histologist
Home Office Pathologist

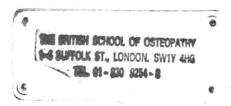
WOLFE MEDICAL PUBLICATIONS LTD

Copyright © G. Austin Gresham, 1971
Published by Wolfe Medical Publications Ltd., 1971
Printed by Smeets-Weert, Holland
SBN 7234 0178 0
5th impression 1984
General Editor, Wolfe Medical Books
G. Barry Carruthers MD (Lond)

This book is one of the titles in the series of
Wolfe Medical Atlases, a series which brings together
probably the world's largest systematic published
collection of diagnostic colour photographs.

For a full list of Atlases in the series, plus
forthcoming titles and details of our surgical, dental
and veterinary Atlases, please write to
Wolfe Medical Publications Ltd, Wolfe House,
3 Conway Street, London W1P 6HE.

Contents

The Concept of Disease

PATHOLOGY is the science of disease. It is concerned with the causes of disease or disorder and the effects of disease-producing agents upon living things, both plants and animals. The ultimate aim of many people who study pathology is the prevention and cure of disease; but first we must study disease as an entity in itself. Only in this way, without the impelling demand to avoid or to treat, can we start impartially to discover mechanisms in the disease producing process.

This atlas is about disease processes, that is to say the various events that appear as disease occurs and progresses. It shows pictures of various tissue and cellular responses to injurious agents. The idea is to lay a foundation of knowledge about fundamental responses that are common to many disorders. When the student has mastered the basic responses he will find no difficulty in understanding special disorders in various systems of the body. For example, inflammation is a basic reaction of many living things to injury of various sorts. Whatever be the cause of inflammation the response and the mechanisms responsible are fundamentally the same.

This, then, is an atlas of general rather than special pathology and is prepared for medical students and other students of biology.

A mole with fungus disease of its lungs is as interesting as a cow with tuberculosis and a man with stomach cancer. Each is a living thing responding to injury. The patterns of response that they exhibit are the subject of our studies in this book.

G. AUSTIN GRESHAM

To my family

Examination of Sections

MOST OF THE WORK that is done in general pathology is concerned with thin, stained sections of tissues rather than with a study of whole organs. The majority are stained with Haematoxylin (blue) and Eosin (red) (H and E); occasionally other stains help to elucidate the nature of the process (special stains).

It is important to have a regular routine for the examination of sections. First look with a hand lens and make a low power drawing. This indicates the need to study different parts of the section. Then turn to the microscope. Most of the useful information can be derived from a study with a low power objective. Higher power lenses are generally less useful except for a study of cell detail.

Having studied the section write a description of it. Whether you can interpret your findings or not is immaterial at this stage. First learn to observe thoroughly and accurately; diagnosis will then come easily and automatically.

Fig. 1. Very low power view of a pituitary to show pink areas of necrosis (cellular death) (H and E x 6)

Fig. 2. Higher power view of a pituitary showing an eosinophilic band of necrotic tissue across the middle of the section (H and E x 45)

Fig. 3. Even higher power view of a necrotic pituitary. Note the loss of nuclear staining in the necrotic area below (H and E x 220)

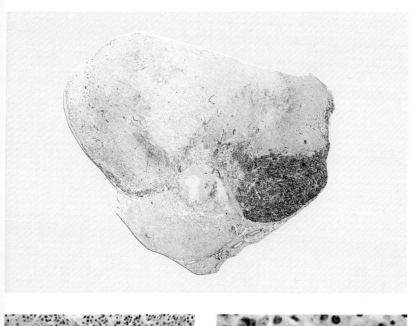

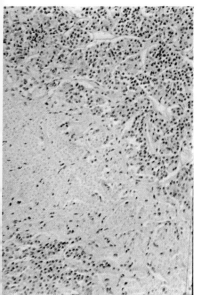

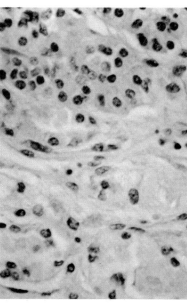

The Lesion

IT IS CONVENIENT to have a general term to describe anything that is wrong with a living thing. The term we use is "lesion"; literally this means a hurting. So we call a fracture of the skull a lesion, a boil on the skin a lesion, a tumour of bone a lesion, and so on. Lesions are often seen with the naked eye; they are said to be macroscopic. Further elucidation of their nature can only be obtained when a thin section is examined under the microscope. Most of this atlas is about microscopic appearances of lesions for only in this way can the precise mechanism of causation be determined.

MACROSCOPIC AND MICROSCOPIC VIEWS OF A LESION

Fig. 4. A slice of left ventricular wall showing grey areas of scarring towards the left side. These are readily visible with the naked eye

Fig. 5. A histological section of a scar in the left ventricular wall showing bright red muscle fibres embedded in pale pink collagenous scar tissue (H and E x 124)

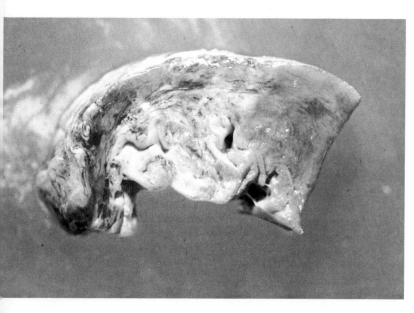

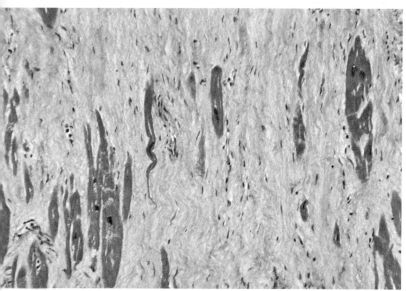

The Normal Cell and Tissue

CELLULAR STRUCTURE

MAMMALIAN CELLS are enormously variable in shape, size and appearance and it is not therefore surprising that diseased cells vary considerably. Yet there are certain features common to many cells; most cells have mitochondria and these are very sensitive to any agent that may damage the cell, except viruses. Mitochondrial damage, therefore, is an early event in cellular disorder. Another general point is that epithelial cells tend to be rather more vulnerable than mesodermal cells. If we look at the edge of a renal infarct (this being an area of necrosis produced by vascular obstruction) we can see dead epithelial cells and surviving fibroblasts of the connective tissue that have withstood the ischaemia.

Another important feature of many epithelial cells is the basement membrane. This supports the cell and also contributes to cellular nutrition. Basement membranes are made of a gelatinous matrix of polysaccharide (mucosubstance) that stains readily with the periodic acid Schiff method (PAS). Reticulin fibres are embedded in the matrix; these fibres are chemically similar to collagen but differ in periodicity when seen by electron microscopy (2·7 nm as against 6·4 nm). They also differ from collagen in being argentaffin; that is, they take up silver salts and are stained black owing to a deposition of metallic silver on them. Reticulin patterns are especially important in diagnostic histopathology of lymph nodes and liver. A disturbance of the pattern, as we shall see later, is an early indication of disease in these organs.

Fig. 6. Kidney showing an area of dead tissue on the left; surviving tissue on the right. This is the edge of a renal infarct (H and E x 50)

Fig. 7. Kidney showing a higher power view of the edge of an infarct. The glomerulus and tubule contain necrotic (pink) cells, but the less specialised spindle shaped fibroblasts have survived and have retained their nuclear staining (H and E x 124)

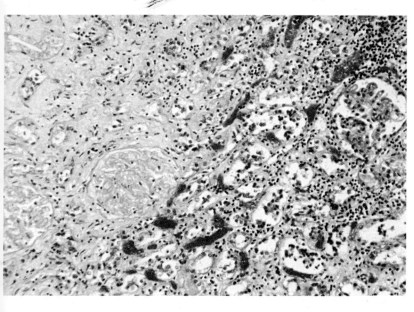

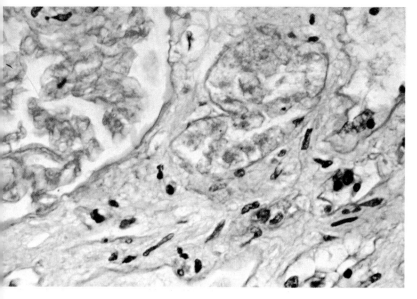

Fig. 8. Normal glomerulus. Note the purple basement membranes of glomerular capillaries and tubules (PAS x 220)

Fig. 9. Normal liver. The cells cannot be seen, but they are outlined by black reticulin basement membranes. Note brown collagen in the portal tract (Gordon and Sweets x 220)

Fig. 10. Reactive centre (so-called germinal follicle) in a lymph node. Note pale central macrophages and peripheral lymphocytes (H and E x 220)

Fig. 11. Reactive centre. Note abundant reticulin fibres around the centre; they are supporting vessels and sinusoids. Normal centres contain few reticulin fibres (Gordon and Sweets x 220)

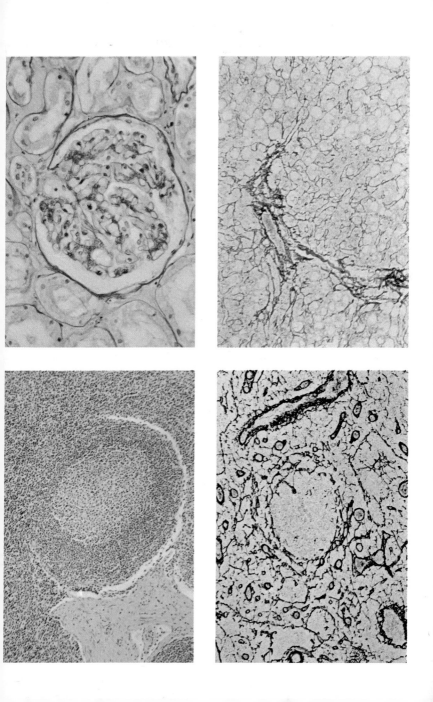

CELLULAR STRUCTURE

Electron Microscopy

The basic ingredients of a cell are shown in the diagram of an electron photomicrograph that follows. There are many variations upon this basic theme. The plasma membrane is thrown into folds (microvilli) in those cells like jejunal and renal proximal tubular cells that are concerned with absorption. Protein-making cells, like plasma cells (*q.v.*), have a rich endoplasmic reticulum studded with ribosomes. Energetic cells have contractile myofilaments or are electrically insulated with coils of myelin in the case of axons of some nerve cells. All cells contain mitochondria, and these are vulnerable to all sorts of injury except viruses; they are the first of the cell organelles to show signs of damage. Lysosomes are bags of hydrolytic enzymes that cause the cell to digest itself (autolysis) or digest other particles (phagocytosis).

Electron microscopy has illuminated the study of cellular disorder mainly by linking organelles with particular functions. This enables the histopathologist to translate morphological alterations into functional disturbances. In some diseases, for example renal glomerular disorders, the only changes that can be detected are demonstrable by the electron microscope; the alterations are far too slight to be detected by light microscopy.

Fig. 12. Diagram of a cell as seen in an electron ▶ micrograph

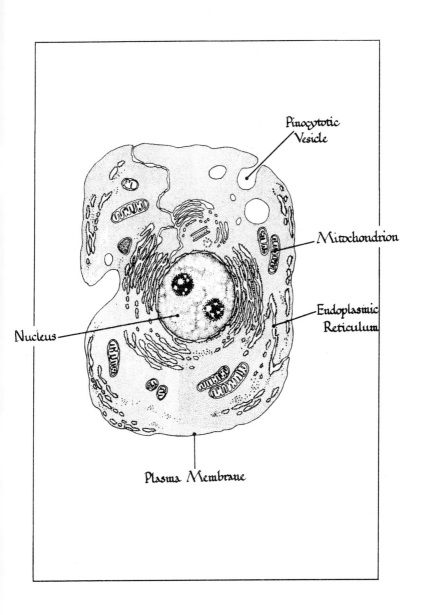

Pinocytotic
Vesicle

Mitochondrion

Endoplasmic
Reticulum

Nucleus

Plasma Membrane

CELLULAR CHEMISTRY
Histochemistry

After ordinary light microscopy, histochemistry is the most often used method for the elucidation of pathological processes. It is an attempt to define chemical constituents of tissue by staining methods that have a clearly defined chemical basis. The earliest of these methods was Perls' for haemosiderin where ferric iron in the tissue combines with potassium ferrocyanide to form Prussian blue.

A variety of histochemical methods is used to show mucin in cells and other polysaccharide in connective tissues. Methods for polysaccharides (mucosubstances) are numerous but not all have a clearly defined basis like Perls' method for ferric iron.

Mucopolysaccharides (mucosubstances) stain by such dyes as mucicarmine and Alcian blue, they are also coloured by the PAS method and by Hale's method.

In Hale's method colloidal iron is made to react with the sulphonic group of the acid mucopolysaccharide and the fixed iron is then demonstrated by Perls' method.

Enzymes in cells and tissues are also demonstrable by histochemical methods. The tissue slice or section is incubated with a substrate; the enzyme acts on the substrate and liberates a component that is made visible in the section either by forming a coloured compound or an insoluble precipitate. For example, alkaline phosphatase is shown by treating a section with glycerophosphate and the liberated phosphate is then treated with cobalt nitrate to produce cobalt phosphate that is finally converted to cobalt sulphide. So the presence of the enzyme is indicated by a black precipitate over and around the cells.

Fig. 13. Heart muscle showing brown pigment in the fibres (H and E x 220)

Fig. 14. Heart muscle stained by Perls' showing that the pigment contains ferric iron (Perls' x 220)

Fig. 15. Colonic mucus-secreting glands. Note the cellular vacuoles that contain mucosubstance (H and E x 350)

Fig. 16. Colonic glands stained by periodic acid Schiff method. This demonstrates neutral mucosubstances. The periodic acid liberates aldehydes from the polysaccharide; these then stain purple with Schiff's reagent (PAS x 350)

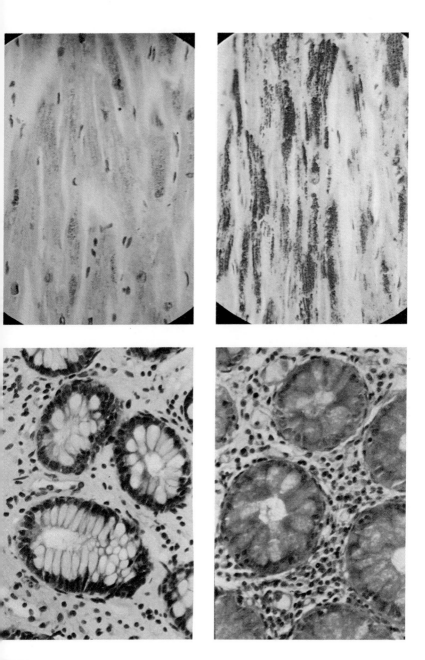

Fig. 17. Colonic glands showing green - staining mucosubstance in the cells (Alcian blue x 350)

Fig. 18. Colonic glands showing blue mucosubstance (Hale x 350)

Fig. 19. Preen gland of bird showing a black luminal border where there is alkaline phosphatase (Gomori x 350)

Fig. 20. Proximal renal tubules of rat showing dense black staining where there is alkaline phosphatase (Gomori x 350)

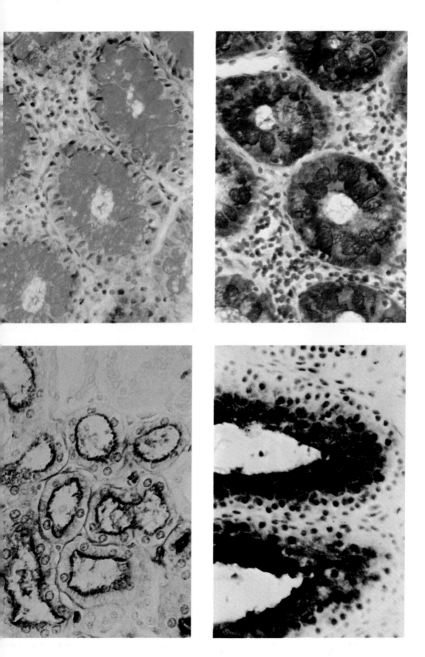

CELLULAR CHEMISTRY
Fluorescence Microscopy

This is another modification of light microscopy which is being used with increasing frequency in histopathology. Briefly, it depends either upon the fact that certain tissue components fluoresce naturally in ultraviolet light (primary fluoresence), or that certain components can be made to fluoresce by treating a section with certain dyes called fluorochromes (secondary fluorescence). Primary fluorescence is shown by elastic fibres after formalin fixation; they are ice-blue when viewed with a microscope using ultraviolet illumination. Fluorochromes are widely used; for example the *Mycobacterium tuberculosis* fluoresces yellow after treatment with auramine O. Because these organisms are often difficult to find in sections or in sputum this method is a valuable, rapid way of detecting them when they are present in small numbers.

Tetracycline is fluorescent and because it is taken up by growing bone it can, when fed to an animal, be subsequently detected in sections of bone viewed in UV light. Yellow areas of tetracycline fluorescence reveal areas of new bone formation and is a valuable adjunct in the study of bone diseases.

S → Sulphur

CELLULAR CHEMISTRY

Autoradiography

Cells take up various elements and compounds and incorporate them into their structure. If these substances are radioactive isotopes then their presence, within the cell, can be shown by autoradiography. Some examples are thyroid cells that take up ^{131} I, dividing cells of all sorts that take up tritiated thymidine and connective tissue cells that incorporate ^{35} S in order to make the mucopolysaccharide matrix.

If an animal is given tritiated thymidine it is taken into cells that are about to divide. If then a section of the tissue is taken and coated with photographic emulsion the cells that contain the label are covered with black dots of silver. This is due to the radiation from the cells, precipitating silver from the photographic emulsion. Hence the mitotic rate can be found.

FLUORESCENCE AND AUTORADIOGRAPHY

Fig. 21. An innominate bone (*left*) and head of humerus (*right*). Note the faint yellow tint of the bones

Fig. 22. Innominate bone and head of humerus viewed in ultraviolet light. Note the bright yellow fluorescence of the tetracycline

Fig. 23. Rat kidney. The black dots are nuclei that have taken up tritiated thymidine. This shows the number of nuclei that are about to divide (Autoradiograph x 500)

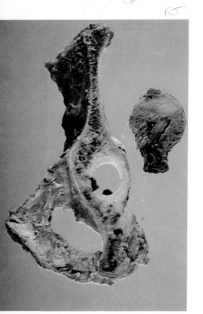
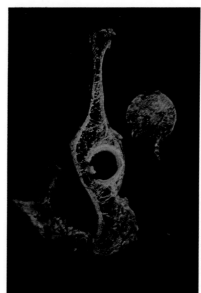
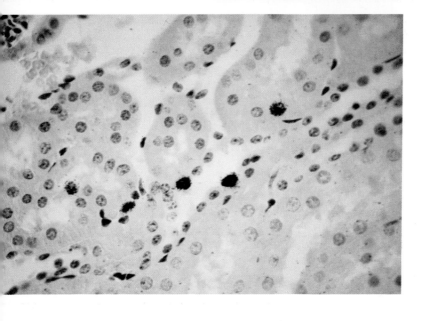

ORGANELLES :- A specialized Part of a cell
that resembles and functions as an
organ.

CELLULAR VARIATION

Cell Types

Cells differ in shape, size, number and distribution of organelles and, of course, in their response to disease-producing agents. For example :—

Nerve cells have abundant R.N.A. (Nissl substance) in their cytoplasm. Loss of this is an early feature of nerve cell damage and is called chromatolysis. This change is reversible when the noxious stimulus is removed.

Plasma cells are protein synthetic and have, in consequence, abundant endoplasmic reticulum. When they are very active, as in many chronic inflammations (*q.v.*) they form intra and extra-cellular aggregates of antibody (Russell bodies).

Mesothelial cells are flat pavement type cells that are barely visible in a transverse section, but when some noxious agent injures the surface such as the pleura or peritoneum the cells swell up and become almost cuboidal in shape. A similar change occurs in synovial cells in many joint conditions. These cells are barely visible in the normal, but any irritation within the joint causes them to swell and become conspicuous.

In the following pages are a few examples of the ways in which cells alter in disease. We shall study many more subsequently.

Eccentric :- not situated in centre.

CELL TYPES

Fig. 24. Neurone. Note purple staining Nissl substance in the cytoplasm of the cell (H and E x 350)

Fig. 25. A group of neurones. Some have lost their Nissl substance (chromatolysis) (H and E x 350)

Fig. 26. A group of plasma cells bordered by collagen (*right*). Note the large red Russell body at the edge of the group of cells. Plasma cells have eccentric nuclei and purple, faintly vacuolated cytoplasm (H and E x 350)

Fig. 27. A cluster of plasma cells. Note the Russell bodies singly and in groups (H and E x 350)

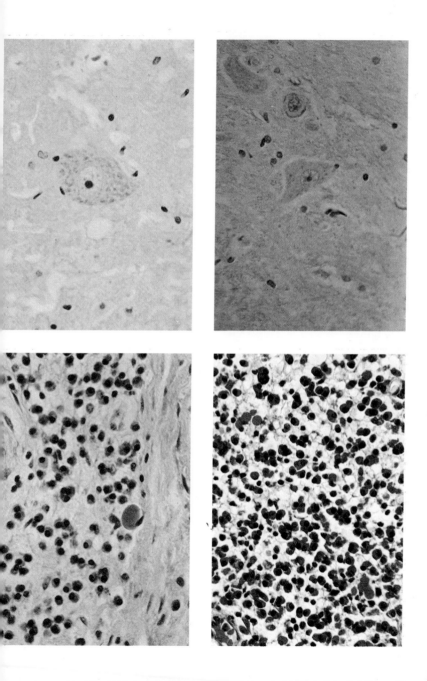

CELL TYPES

Fig. 28. Swollen mesothelial cells (*left*) on the serosal surface of an inflamed vermiform appendix (H and E x 350)

Fig. 29. Slightly swollen synovial cells overlying a cluster of plasma cells from a case of rheumatoid arthritis (H and E x 350)

Fig. 30. Considerably enlarged "irritated" synovial cells. Note the characteristic surface granules that appear in many joint disorders (H and E x 500)

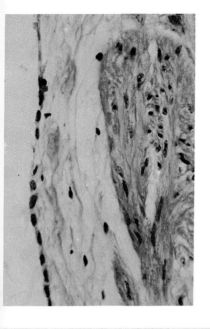
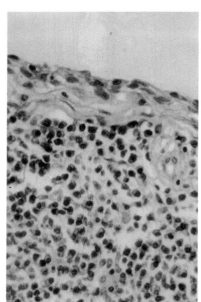
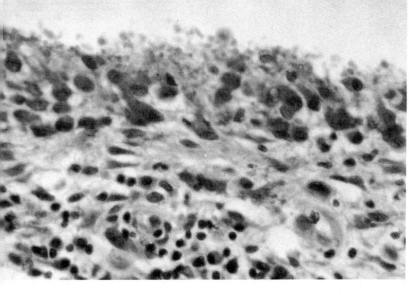

CELLULAR VARIATION

Atrophy

Atrophy is a shrinkage of cells that may be physiological, as in the shrinking uterus after pregnancy, or in the mammary lobules after lactation. It also occurs frequently in disease. For example, in old age or in certain diseases associated with great loss of weight the heart shrinks, the fibres become atrophic and contain much brown pigment called lipochrome (because of its lipoid content) or wear and tear pigment. This pigment is also seen in certain neurones, in liver and in other cells; it is probably derived from fragmented mitochondrial membranes.

Atrophy is caused by hypoxia, disuse of a structure such as a limb or by injurious agents. For example, atrophy of the villi of the small gut is sometimes due to the ingestion of gluten (from bread) in the diet. Such atrophy leads to failure of fat absorption and the production of bulky frothy stools (steatorrhoea). No one knows how gluten acts; when it is removed from the diet the small gut mucosa may return to normal.

Fig. 31. Normal jejunal villi (H and E x 220)

Fig. 32. Atrophic, "flat", jejunal mucosa in gluten dependent enteropathy (H and E x 220)

Fig. 33. Autonomic ganglion cells containing brown lipochrome pigment (H and E x 350)

Fig. 34. Autonomic ganglion cells containing lipochrome pigment staining purple (Gomori's aldehyde fuchsin)

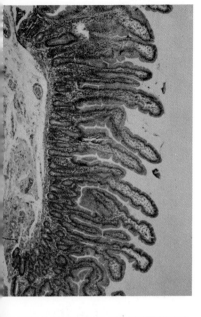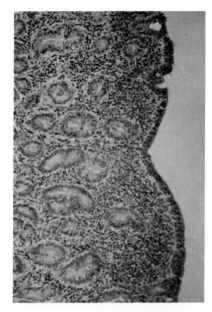
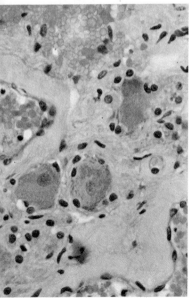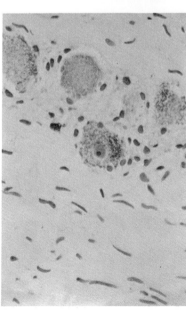

Fig. 35. Brown lipochrome between two nuclei in heart muscle. The pigment often lies close to the nucleus (H and E x 350)

Fig. 36. Abundant purple lipochrome practically obscures the myocardial nuclei (Gomori's aldehyde fuchsin x 350)

Fig. 37. Lipochrome in liver cells. Larger brown globules of bile pigment in canaliculi. From an old person with obstruction of the bile duct (H and E x 350)

Fig. 38. Lipochrome in liver staining purple. Nuclei and bile pigment stain pale blue (Gomori's aldehyde fuchsin x 350)

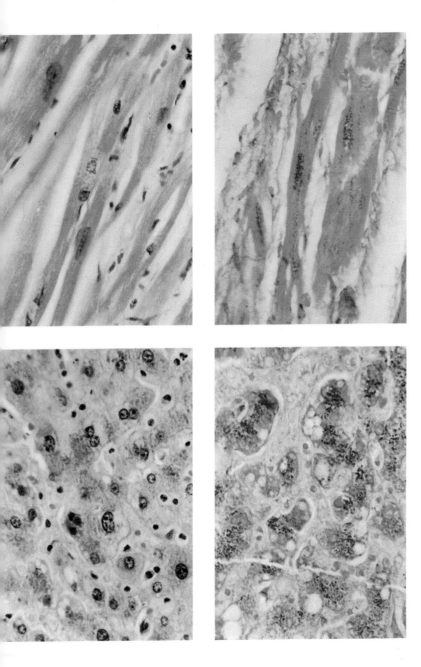

CELLULAR VARIATION

Hypertrophy

This term can be applied both to cells and to organs. Hypertrophy of an organ is a symmetrical increase in size; hypertrophy of a cell is a uniform increase in size of nucleus and cytoplasm. When the organ is required to do more work, the cells hypertrophy. This is readily seen in the myometrial cells of the pregnant uterus; it also occurs in left ventricular myocardial fibres when the arterial blood pressure rises as in hypertensive disease. Unfortunately, hypertrophy is not always accompanied by an increase in blood supply to the enlarged cell. This event is seen in the myocardium; as the fibres get large they become relatively short of blood supply (ischaemia); they then atrophy and are replaced by fibrous tissue (*q.v.*).

HYPERTROPHY

Fig. 39. A low power view of a section of left ventricle from a hypertensive person. Note enlargement of some of the myocardial cells and of their nuclei (H and E x 90)

Fig. 40. A high power view of hypertrophied myocardial fibres. Note that the nuclei are also enlarged (H and E x 350)

Fig. 41. Normal and hypertrophied myocardial fibres near to an ischaemic, fibrotic area. This is compensatory hypertrophy (H and E x 90)

Fig. 42. Broad, thickened hypertrophied epidermis overlying a dermal fibroma (*q.v.*) (H and E x 90)

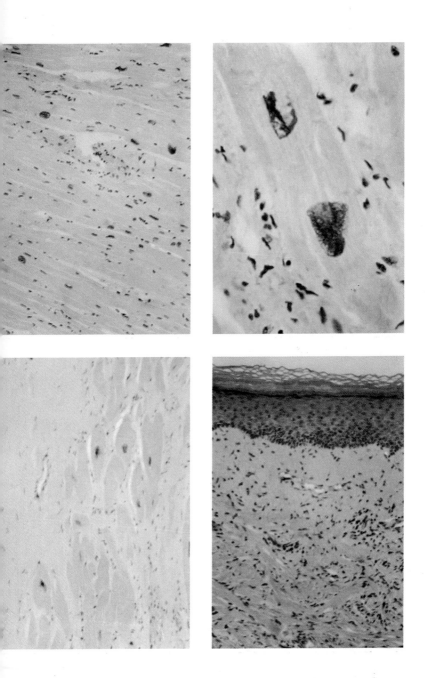

CELLULAR VARIATION
Hyperplasia

This is an increase in the number of cells in a tissue. Hyperplasia is a physiological event in the breast during pregnancy as the cells multiply in order to prepare for lactation after delivery. A similar hyperplasia occurs in the endometrial cells during the menstrual cycle. Hyperplasia is also a pathological process; it occurs in the prostate of elderly men causing the organ to hypertrophy or enlarge. It also occurs as a result of high oestrogen levels, in the elderly female where the cells lining the endometrial glands increase greatly in numbers and size; in other words, there is both hyperplasia and hypertrophy of the cells. Hyperplasia of cells lining the alveoli of the lung is another example of pathological hyperplasia. This phenomenon is called "epithelialisation" of alveoli and is the end result of a wide variety of chronic (longstanding) insults that damage lung tissue. It is, for example a feature of chronic lung infections.

Fig. 43. Hypertrophy of endometrial tubules caused by hyperplasia and hypertrophy of the epithelial cells. From an old lady with hyperoestrogenism (H and E x 220)

Fig. 44. Normal non-secretory endometrial tubules (H and E x 220)

Fig. 45. Hyperplasia of alveolar lining cells in a child with chronic pulmonary infection. Note the normal bronchiole on the left (H and E x 310)

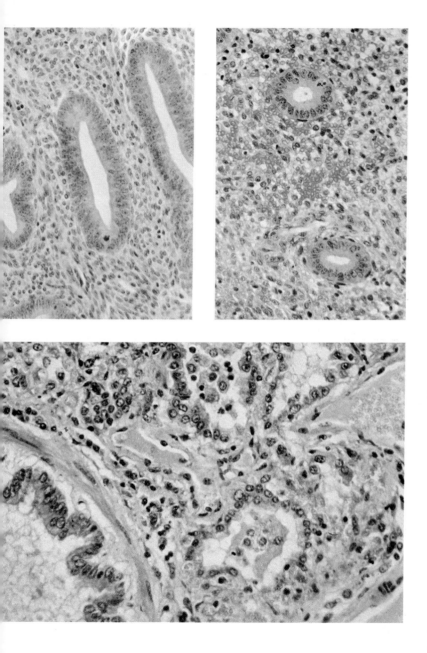

CELLULAR VARIATION
Metaplasia

This is a change in cell character. For example, the transformation of ciliated cells in the bronchi into squamous cells is called squamous metaplasia. It is usually the result of repeated chronic irritation such as smoking and may be the precursor of carcinoma (*q.v.*). Similar squamous metaplasia occurs in the transtional epithelium of the urinary tract caused by irritating hydrocarbons excreted in the urine.

Hormones will sometimes change the character of an epithelium. Squamous metaplasia in the prostate is caused by stilboestrol (a synthetic oestrogen) used for the treatment of prostatic carcinoma (*q.v.*).

Fig. 46. Normal, pseudo-stratified, ciliated, mucus secreting, columnar epithelium of a bronchus (H and E x 350)

Fig. 47. Normal bronchial epithelium showing green droplets of mucosubstance in the cells (Alcian blue x 350)

Fig. 48. Metaplastic bronchial epithelium from a heavy smoker. Note the transformation of the epithelium to a squamous type (H and E x 350)

Fig. 49. Metaplastic bronchial epithelium. Occasional intercellular bridges are present similar to those seen in epidermal cells (Mallory's phosphotungstic acid haematoxylin x 350)

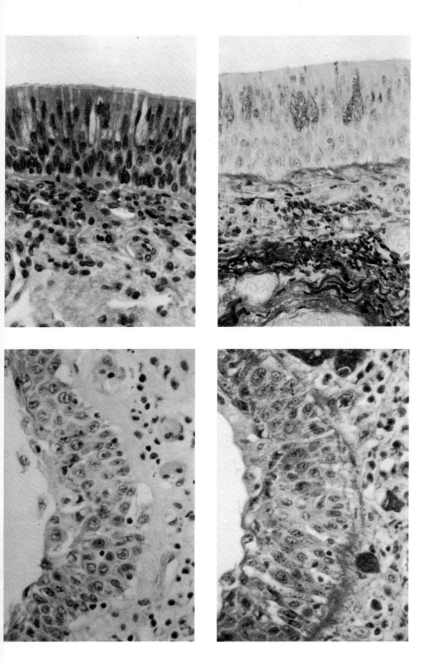

Fig. 50. Normal prostatic acini lined by columnar cells and separated by a fibrous and muscular stroma (H and E x 124)

Fig. 51. A prostatic acinus enlarged and filled with metaplastic, squamous cells. From a man treated with stilboestrol (H and E x 124)

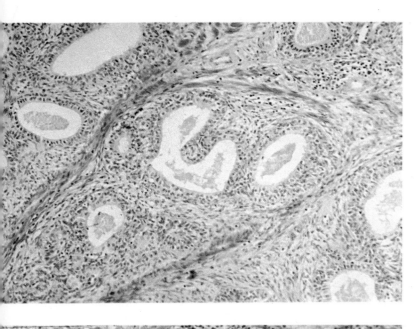

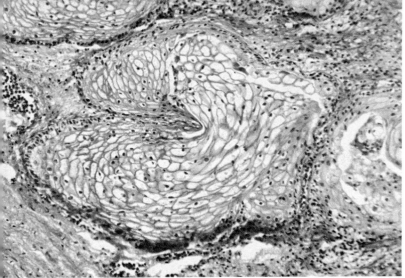

Cellular Damage

SWELLING

CELLULAR SWELLING is the earliest evidence of cellular injury; this is because mitochondria are very vulnerable to noxious agents. When they are damaged cellular metabolism fails and sodium ions enter the cell. This and the osmotic effect caused by the breakdown of large macromolecules within the damaged cell causes cloudy swelling. This is a reversible change and precedes those that are described in the next pages. Macroscopically the organ affected by cloudy swelling is heavier than normal, has a featureless cut surface and bulges from the capsule (*e.g.* liver and kidney). Microscopically the cells are swollen and finely granular; the granules are bits of mitochondria and of other structural proteins

Fig. 52. Cut surfaces of kidneys showing cloudy swelling.
Note the pale swollen cortex and interpyramidal columns

vague

Fig. 53. Hazy, swollen, vacuolated and finely granular
proximal tubular cells in cloudy swelling (H and E x 500)

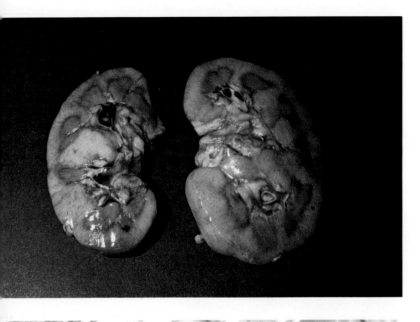
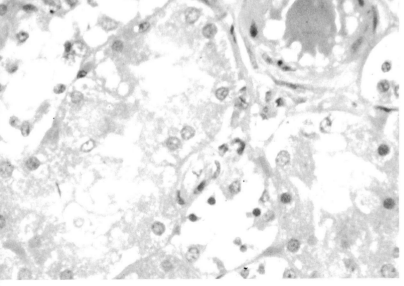

CELLULAR DAMAGE
Vacuolation

Cloudy swelling is the first step of cellular degeneration; the next phase is the appearance of vacuoles in the cytoplasm of the damaged cell; subsequently the cell may die and undergo necrosis. As we have said already, the effects of noxious agents often follow this pattern but do vary according to:—

(1) *The type* of cell affected
(2) *The nature* of the noxious stimulus
(3) *The intensity* of the stimulus
(4) *The duration* of the stimulus.

Considering the first variable, the type of cell. Vacuoloation of liver cells is usually due to the accumulation of fat; so-called fatty change. Vacuolation of renal tubular cells is due to the collection of watery fluid in the cells; so-called hydropic change. Both types of vacuolation are reversible processes. Fatty change in the liver can be due to a variety of noxae:—

(1) *Hypoxia—e.g.* anaemia (*q.v.*)
(2) *Poisons—e.g.* alcohol
(3) *Metabolic* disorder—*e.g.* diabetes mellitus
(4) *Nutritional* deficiency—*e.g.* methionine lack.

However, fatty change must persist for months or even years before the liver cells are irreversibly damaged and are incapable of a return to normal when the damaging agent is removed

Fig. 54. A group of portal liver cells distended with droplets that had contained fat. (This was dissolved in the process of paraffin embedding) (H and E x 220)

Fig. 55. A higher power view of periportal liver cells distended with fat droplets. Periportal fatty change is often due to toxins from gut infections (H and E x 350)

Fig. 56. Centrilobular fatty change. A frozen section shows the red droplets of fat. A variety of poisons (*e.g.* chloroform) may cause this change (Sudan III/IV x 90)

Fig. 57. Subcapsular fatty change in the liver. This is often caused by generalised hypoxia as in anaemia (Phloxine Tartrazine x 90)

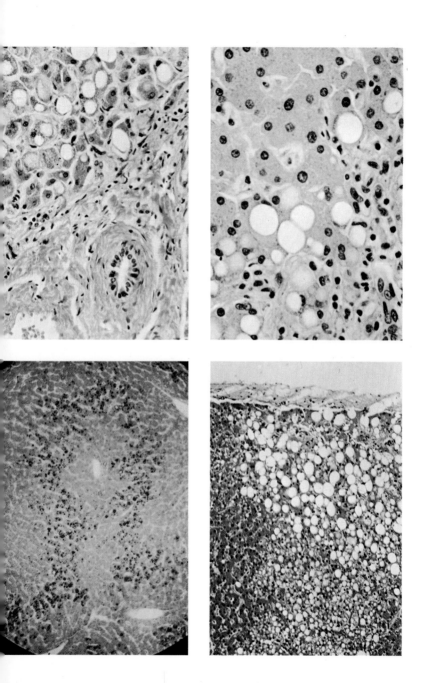

VACUOLATION:
HYDROPIC CHANGE

Fig. 58. Renal tubular cells distended with watery fluid; compare the adjacent normal tubules. Hydropic change in the kidney may be caused by diuretics, hypoxia and a variety of poisons (H and E x 220)

Fig. 59. Hydropic change affecting all the renal tubules in this section. From a man given mannitol to promote a diuresis (H and E x 220)

Fig. 60. Liver showing hydropic change. Note how the cells retain their shape unlike the appearances of fatty change (H and E x 350)

Fig. 61. Heart muscle showing hydropic change in sub-endocardial fibres; these are most susceptible to hydropic change as they are the least well supplied by the coronary circulation (H and E x 220)

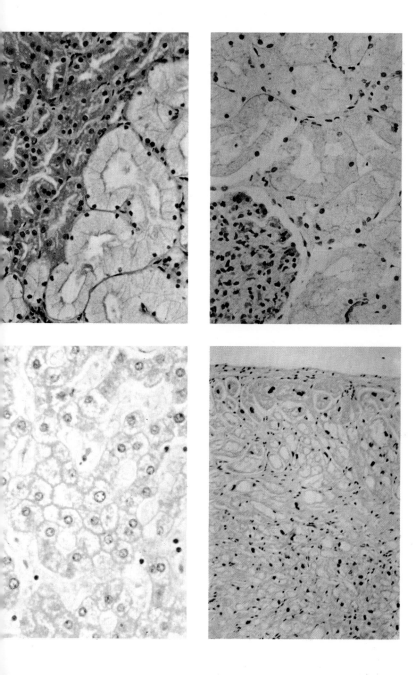

Fig. 62. High power view of heart muscle fibres showing hydropic change. The cells are distended with fluid and the cytoplasm is displaced (H and E x 350)

Fig. 63. Ischaemic skeletal muscle showing hydropic change in a few swollen fibres (H and E x 90)

Fig. 64. High power view of an ischaemic skeletal muscle fibre showing hydropic change at the centre (H and E x 500)

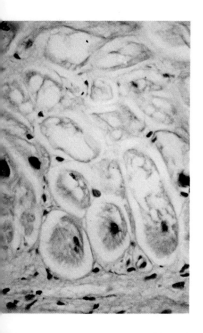

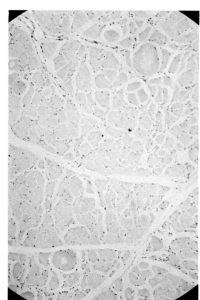

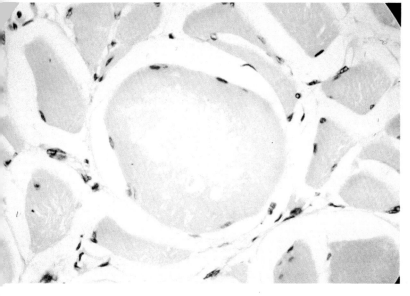

CELLULAR DAMAGE

Accumulations

A variety of substances may collect in cells and in supporting tissues in pathological states. Sometimes the accumulation is of physiological components in excess; for example, iron in the liver, copper in the liver and cornea, glycogen in the liver and, so on. At other times the material that collects is an abnormal metabolite or substance such as amyloid (*q.v.*). Diseases characterised by the appearance of such substances are sometimes called infiltrations; examples of such materials are:—

(1) Mucoid	(5) Hyaline
(2) Lipoid	(6) Iron
(3) Amyloid	(7) Copper
(4) Fibrinoid	(8) Calcium.

Mucoid is a loose term to describe the appearance of mucopolysaccharides in the connective tissue; mucin describes intracellular epithelial polysaccharides as in colonic cells; both are mucosubstances. Mucoid sometimes collects in the aortic wall, giving rise to cystic gaps that weaken the wall and provoke aortic rupture; this is sometimes called aortic medionecrosis. There is a group of diseases called mucopolysaccharidoses where a variety of these substances (mucosubstances) is found in various organs.

Lipoid is found in reticuloendothelial cells of liver, spleen, marrow and other organs. Such disorders are called lipoidoses; various lipoids collect in the different diseases. Lipoidoses are very rare disorders.

Amyloid is a glycoprotein deposited in the perivascular connective tissues of liver, spleen, kidney and adrenal. It occurs in diseases where y globulin levels are persistently high in the blood and can be regarded as a perverted response to protracted antigenic stimulation. In H and E stained sections it is red. It is metachromatic with methyl violet, staining purple red instead of violet, which is the natural colour of the dye. It also stains orange with Congo Red and a variety of colours with other dyes, but no staining method can recognise it specifically.

Fibrinoid and hyaline are eosinophilic materials and resemble one another closely in histological appearance. Hyaline is a clear, glassy, amorphous eosinophilic material that appears in droplets in cells (for example, in renal tubular cells where there is proteinuria) or in the connective tissues as in old scars. Radiation will induce hyalinisation of arteries and so will hypertension; hyaline arteries are also often seen in old people. Fibrinoid is less glassy and more fragmented than hyaline; it is called fibrinoid because it resembles fibrin in its staining appearances. Chemically there are several kinds of fibrinoid so it is not a homogeneous entity.

Metals collect in tissues either because they are present in excess (e.g. copper in Wilson's disease, ferric iron in haemochromatosis and transfusional siderosis of the liver, calcium in hyperparathyroidism), or because they are deposited in dead or dying tissues (e.g. calcium in old scars). These are more accumulations than infiltrations; the material is often found within the cells.

Metastatic calcification is the deposition of calcium when the blood level is high; dystrophic calcification is the deposition of calcium into a dead or dying tissue as in old tuberculous scars or in old arteries when the blood calcium level is normal.

Fig. 65. Aortic wall showing blue staining collections of mucosubstance in Marfan's syndrome (Alcian blue x 100)

Fig. 66. Dissecting aneurysm caused by mucosubstance accumulation; this weakens the vessel wall so that blood dissects through the wall. The original lumen *(left)* is flattened. Blood clot lies between adventitia and outer media (H and E)

Fig. 67. Spleen, Gaucher's disease showing a cluster of lipoid laden cells in the red pulp (H and E x 90)

Fig. 68. Spleen from Gaucher's disease. A thick frozen section showing lipoid in the macrophages in the red pulp (Sudan III/IV x 220)

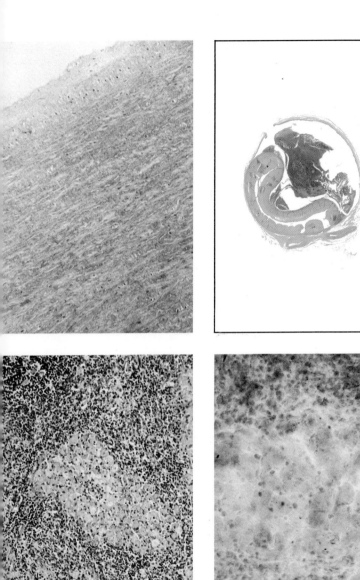

Fig. 69. Masses of pink staining amyloid *(above)* with compressed liver cells *(below)* (H and E x 90)

Fig. 70. A higher power view of hepatic amyloid staining orange-pink (Congo Red x 220)

Fig. 71. A low power view of orange-pink staining amyloid in renal glomeruli. Note the peritubular deposits of amyloid (Congo Red x 90)

Fig. 72. A high power view of extensive infiltration of a glomerulus by purple-red amyloid (Methyl violet x 350)

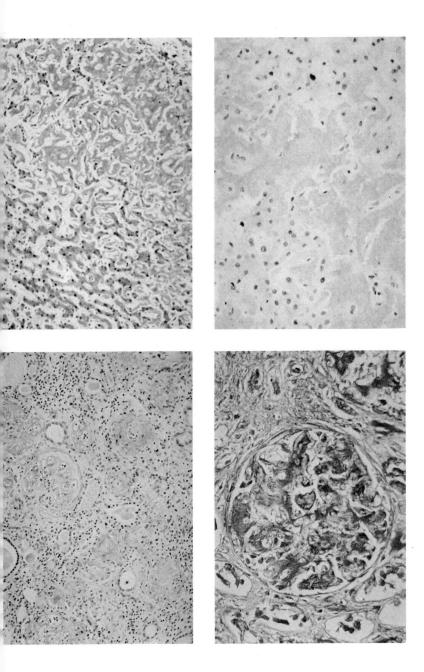

Fig. 73. An afferent renal, glomerular arteriole cut in two planes showing replacement of the wall of the vessel by hyaline material (H and E x 220)

Fig. 74. Pink, glassy, hyaline deposit beneath the endothelium in part of the wall of an afferent glomerular arteriole. This is often seen in hypertensive disease (McFarlane's modification of Mallory's trichrome x 220)

Fig. 75. Hyaline replacement of an artery from an irradiated breast carcinoma (H and E x 90)

Fig. 76. Hyaline replacement of a splenic arteriole. This is a common event that is not related to hypertensive disease (H and E x 90)

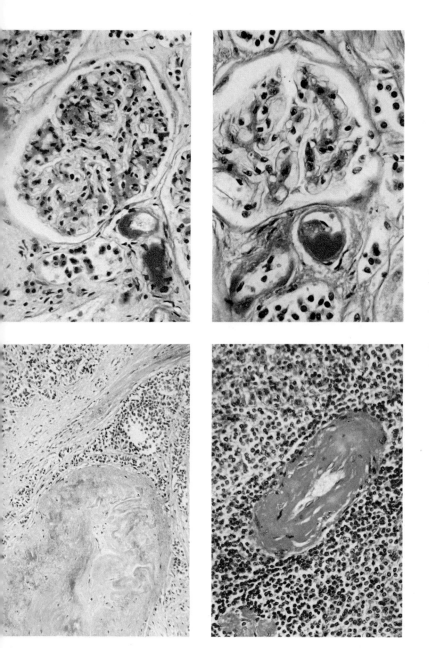

Fig. 77. Hyaline deposits in a glomerulus and in afferent and efferent arterioles of a diabetic. Note the resemblance to amyloid (H and E x 220)

Fig. 78. A nodular collection of hyaline material and diffuse deposits in a glomerulus of a diabetic subject (PAS x 220)

Fig. 79. Hyaline material lining alveoli in the lung of a new born child from a case of respiratory distress syndrome (H and E x 220)

Fig. 80. Hyaline membranes staining blue from a case of respiratory distress syndrome. Lack of pulmonary surfactant is thought to promote undue vascular permeability leading to hyaline membrane formation (McFarlane's modification of Mallory's trichrome)

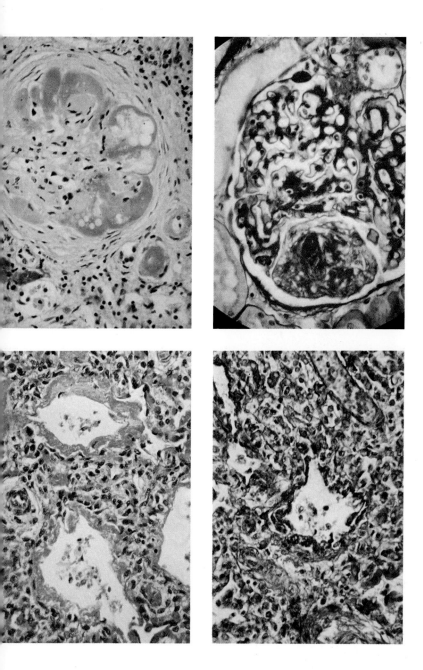

ACCUMULATIONS:
FIBRINOID

Fig. 81. A fringe of synovium *(below)* with an adjacent strip of fibrinoid material enclosing a few fibroblast nuclei. From a case of rheumatoid arthritis (H and E x 350)

Fig. 82. Clumps of eosinophilic fibrinoid material in a chronic inflammatory exudate *(q.v.)* on the pericardium (H and E x 220)

Fig. 83. Fibrinoid material *(above)* in the wall of a chronic peptic ulcer of the stomach (H and E x 90)

Fig. 84. A strip of fibrinoid material bordered by a palisade of macrophages in a rheumatoid granuloma *(q.v.)* (H and E x 220)

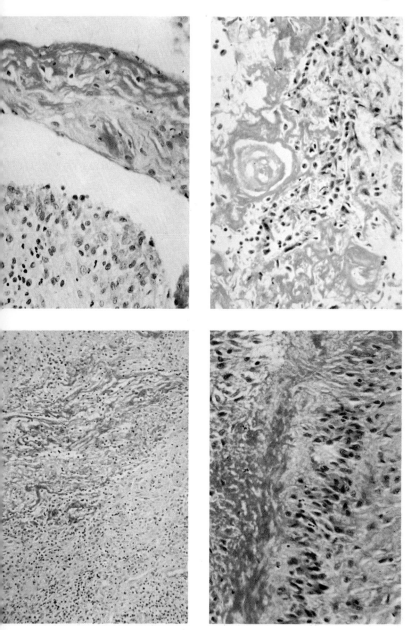

Fig. 85. Brown, iron-containing haemosiderin in liver and Kupffer cells from a patient who had received many transfusions (H and E x 350)

Fig. 86. Blue staining haemosiderin from a case of transfusional siderosis. The iron is deposited because of haemolysis (Perls' x 350)

Fig. 87. A thin black line of copper *(left)* in Descemet's membrane from a case of Wilson's disease (Rubeanic acid x 350)

Fig. 88. Black deposits of calcium in old eosinophilic scar tissue (H and E x 220)

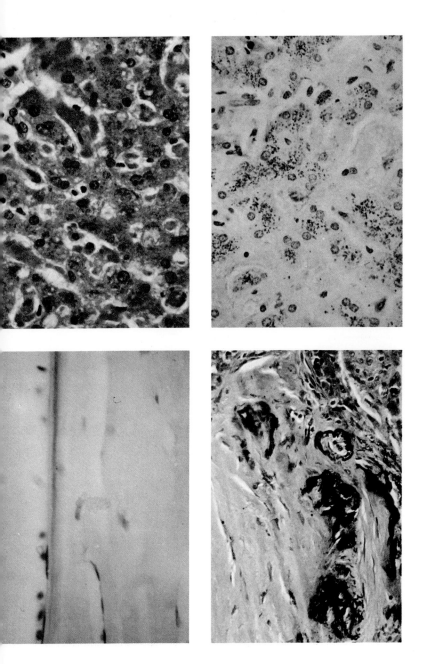

Fig. 89. Black deposits of calcium between myocardial fibres. Metastatic calcification from a case of hyperparathyroidism (H and E x 124)

Fig. 90. Blue deposits of haemosiderin· in cerebral arterioles from the region of an old cerebral infarct (*q.v.*) (Perls' x 124)

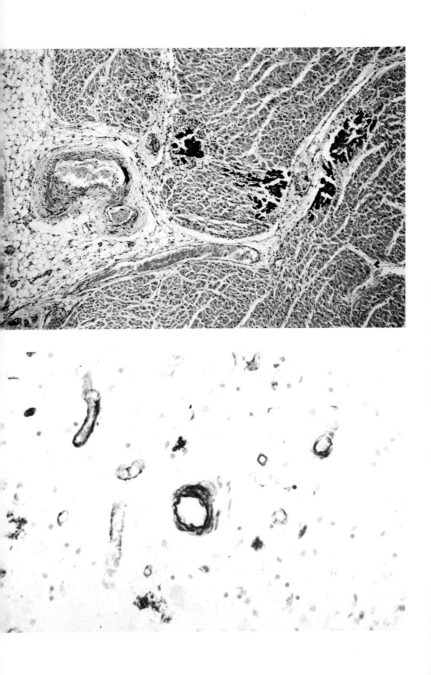

Irrevocable := Can not be "called back"
or "cancelled".

CELLULAR DAMAGE

Autolysis

This is an irrevocable affair. Hydrolytic enzymes are released from cells in which the lysosomal membranes have broken down ; then the cell virtually digests itself. Autolysis occurs post mortem as a usual event in the breakdown of the body. Before death it is the late result of cell injury. It is often difficult to distinguish post mortem from ante mortem autolysis, but nuclear changes tend to be severe if the cell has been injured during life.

Autolysis is more conspicuous in some organs than others. It is commonly seen in the gut and in other glandular organs such as pancreas, kidneys and suprarenals.

CELLULAR DAMAGE

Necrosis

This means death of a cell or tissue. Necrotic changes are made up of cytoplasmic alterations (which we have already described) and nuclear changes that are:

(1) *Pyknosis*—intense nuclear shrinkage, often seen in intense damage *e.g.* burning of a tissue;
(2) *Karyolysis*—where the nucleus swells up and lyses;
(3) *Karyorhexis*—here the nucleus breaks into fragments. Such fragments are commonly seen in reactive centres in lymph nodes.

So far we have described the microscopical appearances of necrosis, but necrotic tissue is also seen macroscopically and presents a variety of different appearances.

(1) *Coagulative* necrosis where the tissue retains its shape but is dead *e.g.* a renal infarct (*q.v.*);
(2) *Liquefactive* necrosis, as in the brain, where the dead tissue liquefies and forms a cyst;
(3) *Caseous* necrosis caused by the *Myco. tuberculosis;* the consistency is soft and cheesy due to lipoids from the organism;
(4) *Gaseous* necrosis (gas gangrene) where bacteria (Clostridia) kill muscle and ferment the glycogen to produce gas bubbles;
(5) *Gummatous* necrosis or rubbery necrosis, where fibrous tissue replacement keeps pace with cell destruction as in syphilis;
(6) *Fat necrosis*—here omental and other fat becomes necrotic and opaque due to the liberation of fatty acids by lipases from a diseased pancreas (pancreatitis).

Fig. 91. Renal tubular cells from a kidney taken within a few hours of death. Early autolytic breakdown of the cytoplasm is present (H and E x 350)

Fig. 92. Severe proximal tubular autolysis from a kidney taken 48 hours post mortem. Note the angular fragmentation of the cells. Glomerulus and distal tubules are fairly well preserved (H and E x 220)

Fig. 93. Severe necrosis of liver around a central vein. Note the loss of cellular outlines and of nuclear staining (H and E x 90)

Fig. 94. Proximal tubular necrosis. Note the total destruction of eosinophilic cells (H and E x 220)

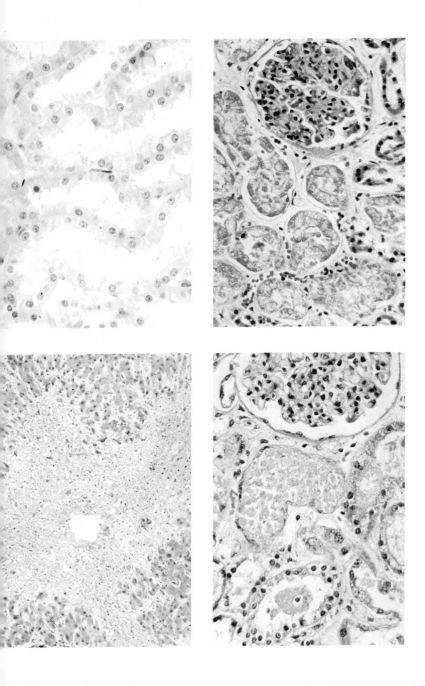

NECROSIS

Fig. 95. Necrotic renal tubules above, normal tubules below. Note the total loss of nuclear staining (H and E x 90)

Fig. 96. Necrotic debris showing shrunken and fragmented nuclei scattered in the amorphous material (H and E x 220)

Fig. 97. A necrotic seminiferous tubule from an infarct (*q.v.*) caused by torsion. Note the ghostly outlines of the spermatogenic cells and the pyknotic and karyorhetic nuclei (H and E x 350)

Fig. 98. Pyknosis and karyolysis in the normal superficial layers of the skin (H and E x 350)

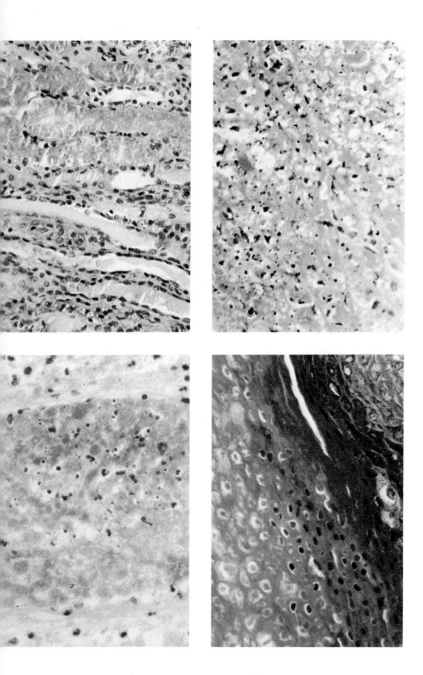

Fig. 99. Recent myocardial necrosis at the edge of an infarct. Note the brightly eosinophilic dead muscle below; granulation tissue above (*q.v.*) (H and E x 90)

Fig. 100. Eosinophilic necrotic skeletal muscle bordered by fibroblasts (H and E x 90)

Fig. 101. A very low power view of cerebellum showing a hole due to liquefactive necrosis (Sudan Black B x 5)

Fig. 102. Pink, caseous necrosis at the centre of tuberculous follicles (*q.v.*). The necrotic area is bordered by mononuclear and giant cells (*q.v.*) (H and E x 90)

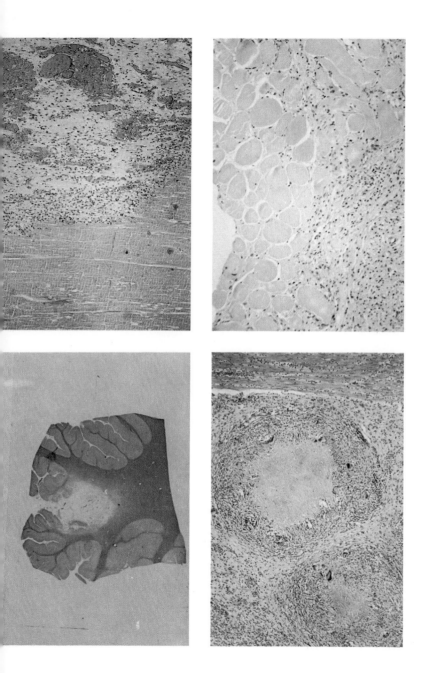

Fig. 103. Liver showing a few relatively normal cells below; the rest are necrotic and show karyolysis (H and E x 220)

Fig. 104. Fat necrosis. Normal cells (*below*) are separated from the featureless necrotic cells (*above*) by a band of cellular infiltrate (H and E x 90)

Fig. 105. Gas gangrene. Necrotic skeletal muscle fibres, on the left, separated by gas and a fibrinous inflammatory exudate (*q.v.*) on the right (H and E x 220)

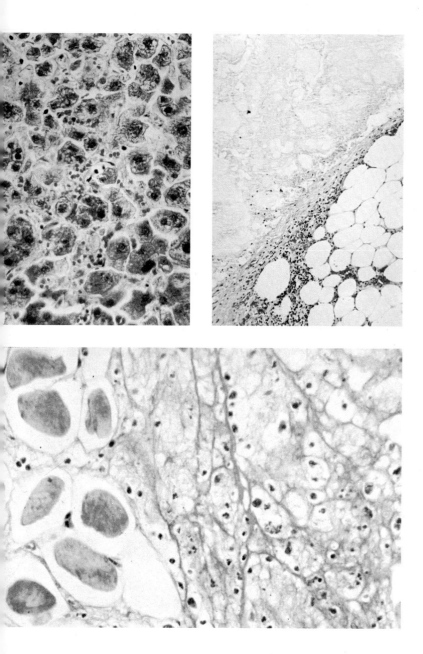

Causes of Cellular Damage

WE DO NOT KNOW the causes of the two main killing diseases of Western man, *viz.* obliterative arterial disease (*q.v.*) and neoplasia (colloquially called cancer) (*q.v.*). A lot is known of infectious agents; although they have been suppressed by hygienic measures in civilised countries they still represent, the world over, the main cause of death and illness.

ANIMATE AGENTS

Virus, Rickettsia, Mycoplasma

They vary greatly in size. At one end fo the scale are the obligate intracellular agents like viruses and rickettsiae, and at the other are large tapeworms occupying much of the small gut.

Virus diseases are common and sometimes, like influenza, notorious. Many viruses produce inclusion bodies in the cells they infect. The appearances of the inclusion and its position (whether in the nucleus or cytoplasm or both) gives a clue to the nature of the infection. For example, the cytomegalovirus of the herpes group enlarges the nucleus with its inclusion producing an owl's eye appearance.

Rickettsiae are also intracellular. The group of arthropod borne diseases now includes others such as ornithosis, trachoma and cat-scratch disease that were once thought to be viruses.

Mycoplasmas resemble the L (Lister) forms of bacteria. They are ubiquitous and are associated with a variety of diseases of man and animals. Mycoplasmal pneumonia is so common in the pig as to be almost a usual finding at slaughter. The lesions are characteristic but the organism, like the rickettsiae, is difficult to find in sections.

Fig. 106. Molluscum contagiosum; a virus-induced lesion of skin. Note the dark staining clusters of inclusion bodies in the epithelial cells (H and E x 35)

Fig. 107. Skin showing inclusion bodies in the common virus wart. The bodies are pink in the stratum granulosum and more blue nearer the surface (H and E x 350)

Fig. 108. A proximal renal tubule showing cytomegalovirus. Note the considerable enlargement of the cells and the basophilic intranuclear inclusions (H and E x 350)

Fig. 109. "Owl's eye" intra nuclear inclusion of cytomegalovirus. This virus is a common opportunist infective agent in patients receiving immunosuppressive drugs. (H and E x 880)

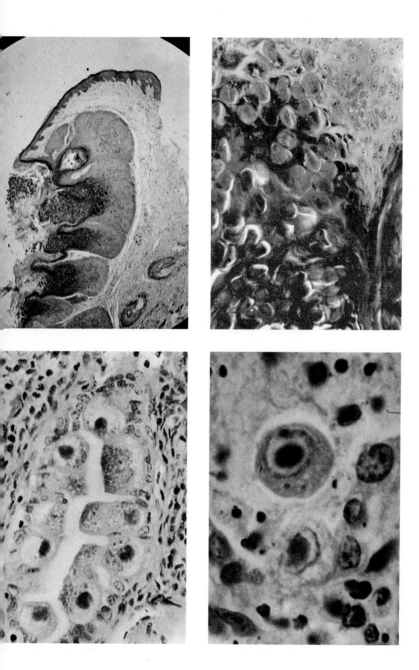

Fig. 110. Bands of pink necrosis in a lymph node from cat-scratch disease. The agent is classed as a rickettsia and is transmitted by cats (H and E x 35)

Fig. 111. A higher power view of cat-scratch disease showing an area of necrosis. in a lymph node, bordered by macrophages (H and E x 90)

Fig. 112. Lung; chronic mycoplasmal pneumonia showing numerous lymphoid follicles near to a bronchiole. This is a characteristic appearance of the late stage of the disease (H and E x 50)

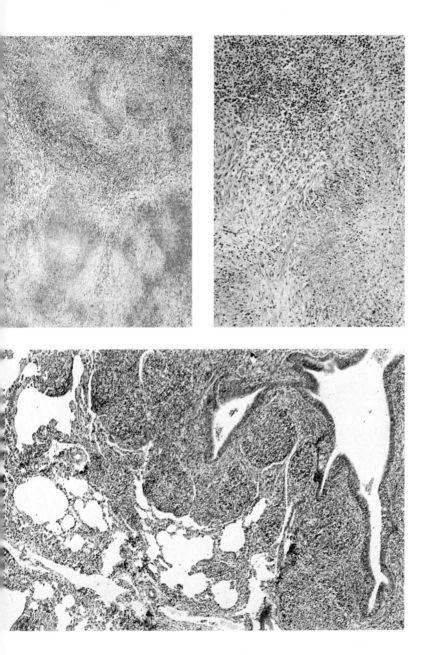

ANIMATE AGENTS

Bacterium and Fungus

Bacteria can often be seen in sections of diseased tissues stained by Gram's method. Some appear as black dots or clumps. They can be readily distinguished from coal dust or other artefact by their regular shape and size.

Fungi are often difficult to see as they stain weakly basophilic with H and E. A PAS or other special stain, such as a silver method, reveals them clearly, however. It is important to think of a possible fungal cause when faced with a section of an obscure chronic inflammation. A PAS stain will rapidly reveal the solution to the problem.

ANIMATE AGENTS: BACTERIUM

Fig. 113. Severe haemorrhagic staphylococcal pneumonia. The organisms appear as a black fringe at the edge of the exudate (H and E x 220)

Fig. 114. Haemorrhagic staphylococcal pneumonia. The layer of organisms stains darkly (Gram x 220)

Fig. 115. Carbon pigment outlining alveoli in the lung. The particles are of variable shape and size and need to be differentiated from bacteria (H and E x 220)

Fig. 116. *Mycobacterium tuberculosis:* clusters of beaded red bacilli in an area of tuberculous necrosis (Ziehl Neelsen x 880)

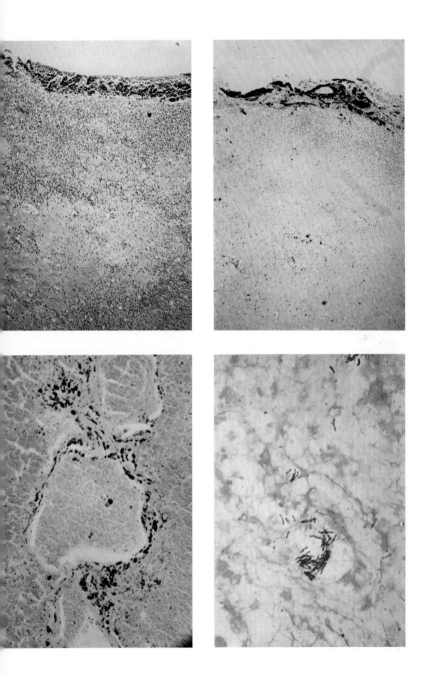

Fig. 117. A group of macrophages in a lesion from a leper. Faint cytoplasmic striations are all that can be seen of the organism (H and E x 880)

Fig. 118. Sheaves of pale pink *Myco. leprae* in macrophages (Modified Ziehl Neelsen x 880)

Fig. 119. Anthrax bacilli in pulmonary capillaries (Gram x 880)

Fig. 120. Anthrax bacilli in hepatic sinusoids from fatal anthrax (Gram x 880)

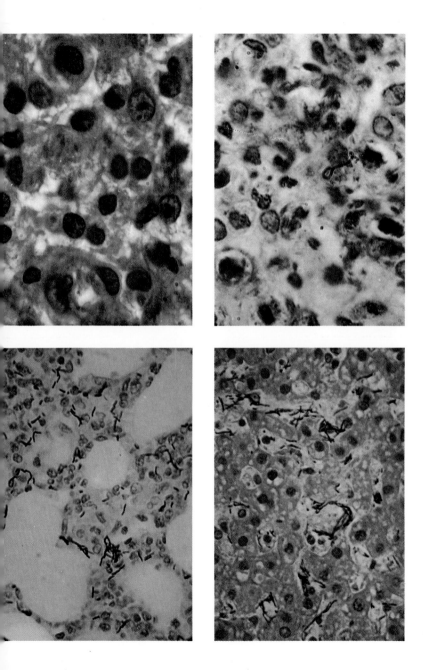

Fig. 121. A group of autolysed liver cells with bacteria in the sinusoids. This is a common post mortem effect and must not be confused with infection (H and E x 350)

Fig. 122. An area of necrosis in the lung containing black fungal hyphae (H and E x 90)

Fig. 123. A higher power view showing red staining, branching fungal hyphae of *Aspergillus sp.* (PAS x 220)

Fig. 124. A clump of aspergillary hyphae in the lung stained by a silver method (Grocott x 350)

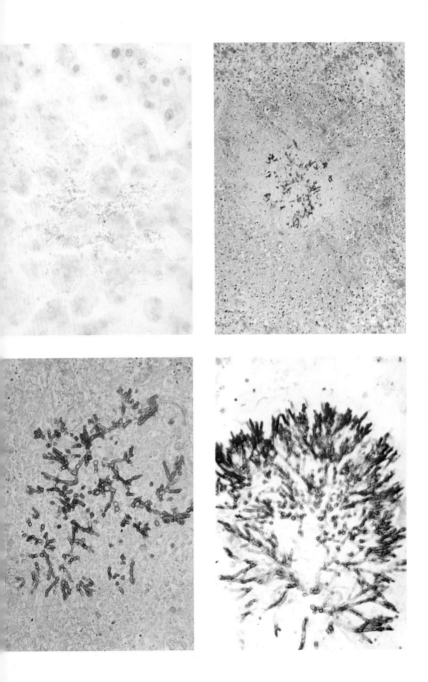

Fig. 125. An area of necrosis (*above*) in the oesophagus of a leukaemic patient (H and E x 90)

Fig. 126. Another section of oesophageal necrosis showing purple threads of the fungus *Candida albicans* (PAS x 90)

Fig. 127. Pale blue spheroidal fungi in a chronic lung abscess (H and E x 220)

Fig. 128. Another section of the lung abscess stained to show the mucosubstance capsule of the fungus (*Cryptococcus neoformans*) (Alcian blue x 220)

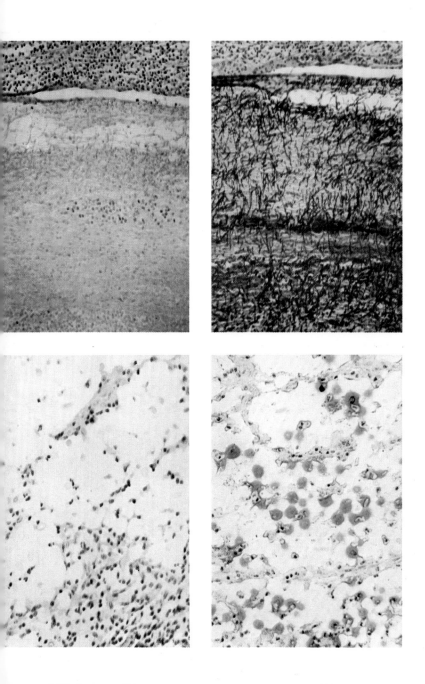

Fig. 129. *Cryptococcus neoformans* in a lung abscess (Gram x 350)

Fig. 130. *Cryptococcus neoformans* in a lung abscess (Alcian blue x 350)

Fig. 131. Brown flask-like fragments of fungus from a case of chromoblastomycosis (H and E x 350)

Fig. 132. A giant celled reaction (*q.v.*) around the causative organism of chromoblastomycosis (*Phialophora sp.*) (H and E x 220)

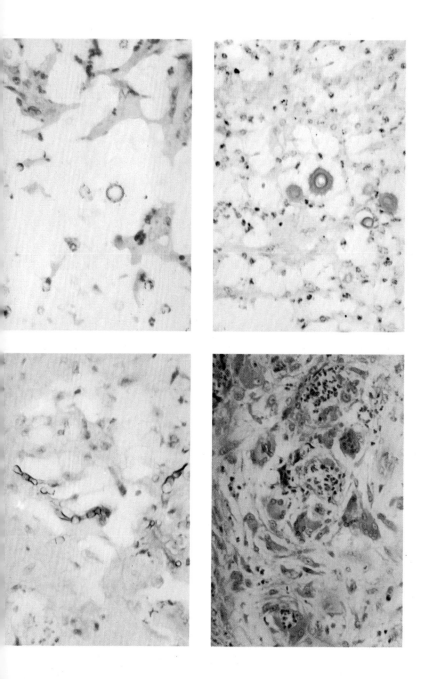

ANIMATE AGENTS

Protozoon

Malaria is a protozoal disease that causes much disease the world over. However, this and other protozoal disorders are uncommon in Western temperate countries for a variety of reasons. A recent small increase in protozoal infections has occurred in Britain because of the use of immunosuppressive agents to enable transplanted organs to survive in a foreign host. These drugs, like azothioprine, damp down the response to foreign proteins and also to most micro-organisms including cytomegalovirus, fungi and protozoa. Some of the latter are sporozoa such as *Toxoplasma gondii* and *Pneumocystis carinii* that may be found in abundance in the lungs and other tissuss of persons dying after organ transplantation.

Fig. 133. A cyst containing boat-shaped sporozoa in skeletal muscle. This protozoon (*Sarcocystis sp.*) is a common incidental finding in animals (H and E x 350)

Fig. 134. Free and encysted *Toxoplasma gondii* in the brain of a person dying with Hodgkin's disease (H and E x 350)

Fig. 135. A higher power view of a cyst in the brain containing toxoplasms (H and E x 880)

Fig. 136. Black staining *Pneumocystis carinii* in alveoli of the lung (Grocott x 660)

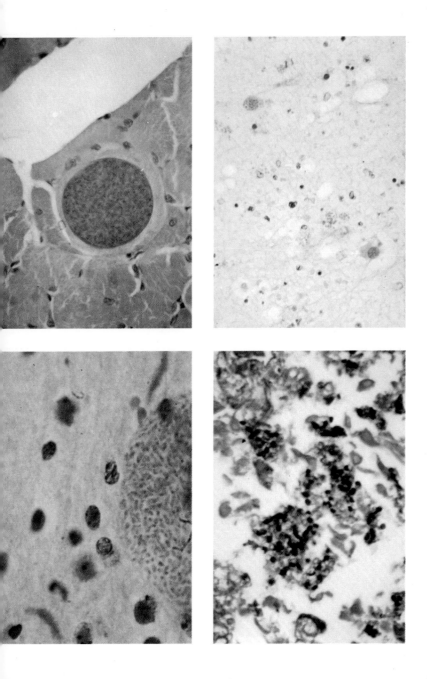

ANIMATE AGENTS

Metazoon

Medical men in this country are, in general, unaware of the possibility of fungal, protozoal and metazoon infections; yet the latter, like the former two can cause serious disease. Metazoa include a diverse range of parasites; many of them are helminths (worms). Some, like tapeworms and pin worms (*Cestoda* and *Nematoda*), are trivial infections. Some, like the liver flukes (*Trematoda*), form the most widespread of world diseases with a high morbidity rate.

Particularly serious are the migrating larvae of certain ascarid worms (*Toxocara canis* and *cati*). These come from dogs and cats; the worms are swallowed by children and the larvae migrate through the tissues (visceral larva migrans). Some of them finish up in the eye and cause a reaction that leads to blindness. In this country toxocariasis is one of the common causes of blindness in children.

Fig. 137. A transverse section of the nematode *Enterobius vermicularis* in the lumen of the vermiform appendix (H and E x 220)

Fig. 138. *Schistosoma mansoni* in the submucosa of the colon. Note the inflammatory reaction (*q.v.*) around the nematodes (H and E x 90)

Fig. 139. Extensive intra-alveolar haemorrhage in association with migratory nematode larvae (visceral larva migrans) (H and E x 90)

Fig. 140. A larva of *Ascaris lumbricoides* in a pulmonary vessel (H and E x 220)

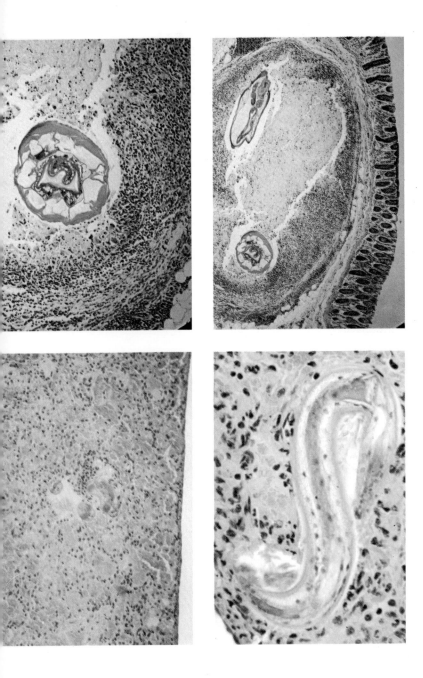

INANIMATE AGENTS

Heat Radiation Poison

The environment is bristling with potentially dangerous agents of all kinds; radiations, dusts and smokes, preservatives in food, drugs and poisons. Some people are more exposed than others; for example, workers with asbestos, silica, cotton dust and so on are likely to develop disease as a result of inhalation of these agents.

Sections of diseased tissues sometimes reveal the cause; *e.g.* iron-coated asbestos particles may be seen in a section of fibrotic lung. Often the cause is not apparent.

Radiation affects tissues either by stimulating cell division or, if the dose is large enough, by killing cells. It also acts more subtly by causing a progressive swelling of arterial walls leading to vascular occlusion and ischaemia. Radiations act at a molecular level, either by scoring "hits" on nuclear D.N.A. or by producing toxic ionic products of water that damage cells.

Poisons is a generic term for a wide range of agents. Some act subtly by interfering with intermediary metabolism (*e.g.* carbon monoxide or fluoracetate), others are crude corrosive agents like the acids and alkalis that destroy cells. Often the poisons tend to act on specific cells like the diphtheria toxin on certain neurones, the aflatoxin (from *Aspergillus flavus*) on the liver, strychnine on the anterior spinal cord neurones, and so on.

Vascular tissues seem to be especially prone to a number of toxic agents. One of the more interesting group of these are alkaloids from plants that form the basis of Jamaican bush tea. These substances cause intimal proliferation of veins and probably in the endocardium of the heart also. The venous intimal proliferation is especially seen in the liver where vessels become occluded throughout the organ. This is so-called veno-occlusive disease.

123

Fig. 141. A cluster of asbestos bodies in an alveolus in the lung. They are brown because they are coated with iron (H and E x 350)

Fig. 142. Blue asbestos bodies coated with iron (Perls' x 350)

Fig. 143. A cluster of asbestos bodies and carbon pigment in an area of pink fibrous tissue in the lung (H and E x 350)

Fig. 144. Areas of blue fibrous thickening of alveolar walls in Paraquat (weedkiller) poisoning (McFarlane's modification of Mallory's trichrome x 220)

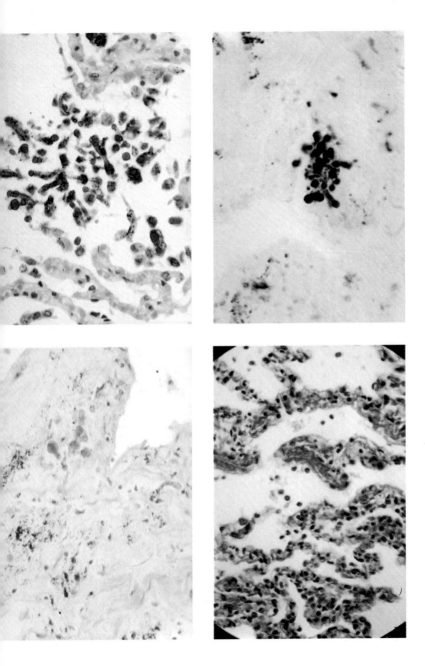

Fig. 145. Irradiated kidney showing many pale-pink sclerotic glomeruli (H and E x 124)

Fig. 146. Irradiated kidney showing many sclerotic glomeruli (Hart's modification of Weigert's stain x 124)

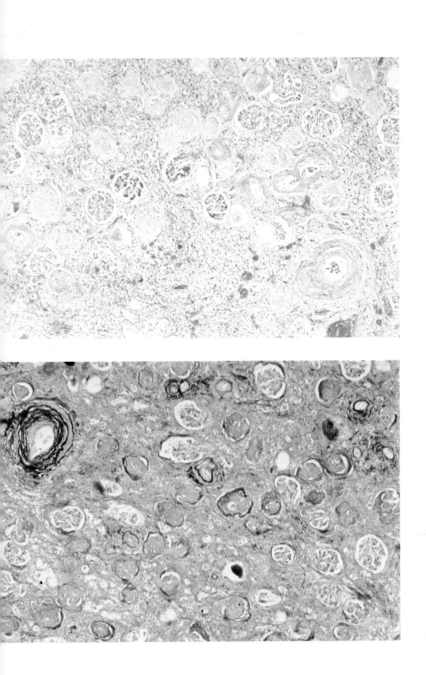

Responses to Cellular Damage

THIS IS PROBABLY the most important chapter in this book, for it illustrates the basic responses of living things when they are injured, whatever the injurious agent may be.

The reactions are local ones at or near the portal of entry of the agent and general reactions may occur throughout the body; these come into play when the disease-producing stimulus is strong enough to elicit the general reaction.

If a staphylococcus enters a hair follicle in the skin surface it provokes an inflammation in the skin that may prevent the organism from spreading. If, however, the organism spreads it does so by lymphatics to the regional lymph nodes where the phagocytic cells of the reticulo-endothelial system multiply. This mechanism may also fail so that the organisms enter the blood stream. This creates a general response composed of fever, a rise in the white blood count (leucocytosis), and a steady rise in the level of antibody globulins derived from lymphoid cells. The role of fever and its cause is still obscure. Leucocytosis might be envisaged as providing more phagocytic cells for the ingestion and destruction of the organism. Antibodies, when they appear, are opsonic; that is to say they promote phagocytosis amongst other actions that they have.

If all fails then *septicaemia* results. The bacteria multiply in the blood stream and the host may die; however, *bacteraemia* is a state where bacteria are present in the blood but growth is arrested by the suppressant effect of antibodies. *Pyaemia* is a grave event where dividing bacteria and particles of necrotic material gain entry to the blood, usually via a vein in the wall of a necrotic zone of tissue. Here, then, are two deadly effects: toxin production by bacteria and ischaemia caused by vascular blockage by necrotic debris.

Phagocytes are microphages (polymorphonuclear neutrophils) and macrophages (variously called monocytes, histiocytes, littoral cells, Kupffer cells, etc.). Antibodies aid their action and they form the most potent deterrent in bacterial infections.

Eosinophil leucocytes sometimes appear in large numbers especially in helminth infections and in allergic disorders. They are phagocytic but their precise role in these conditions remains to be elucidated.

Thrombocytosis is a rise in the platelet count of the blood. This is a delayed response taking a few days to develop and often follows extensive trauma or splenectomy. It might be envisaged as a protective mechanism to encourage thrombosis in blood vessels (*q.v.*) thereby preventing bleeding that might occur after tissue damage.

Fig. 147. A blood film showing many polymorphonuclear neutrophil leucocytes in this high power field (leuco-cytosis). Note that they are young polymorphonuclear cells with few lobes on the nuclei (Leishman x 1200)

Fig. 148. A blood film showing a polymorphonuclear neutrophil leucocyte together with many blue-staining platelets (thrombocytosis). Some of the platelets are rather large (Leishman x 1200)

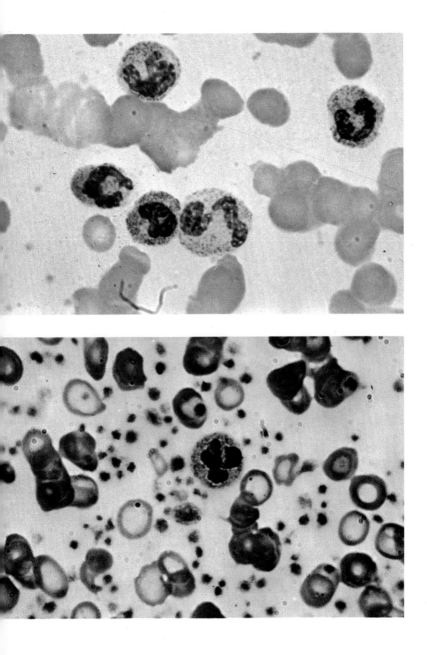

Fig. 149. Reactive centres in the cortex of a lymph node. The pale centres are composed of macrophages (H and E x 90)

Fig. 150. High power view of the edge of a reactive centre. The large pale cells are macrophages. Note the rows of lymphocytes at the edge ; this is a characteristic feature of a reactive centre (H and E x 350)

Fig. 151. Proliferation of sinus-lining macrophages (littoral cells) in a sinus of a lymph node (H and E x 220)

Fig. 152. Phagocytosis of injected carmine by littoral cells in a guinea pig (H and E x 350)

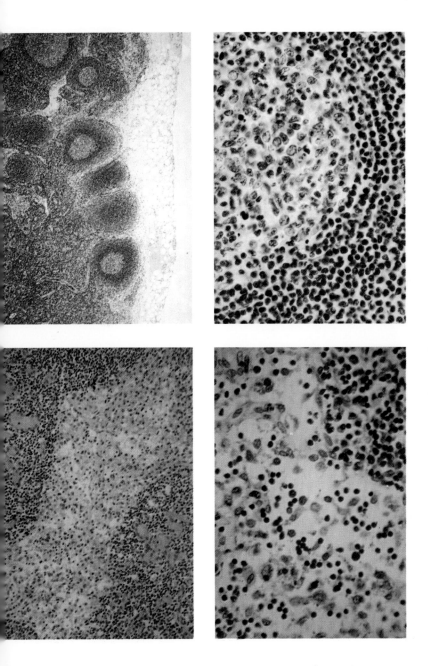

Fig. 153. Phagocytosis of coal dust by macrophages in a bronchial lymph node (H and E x 90)

Fig. 154. Lipoid laden phagocytic microglial cells at the edge of necrotic brain tissue. These bloated cells are called Gitterzellen or compound granular corpuscles (H and E x 350)

Fig. 155. Smear of gonococcal pus showing intracellular cocci in polymorphonuclear leucocytes (Gram x 1200)

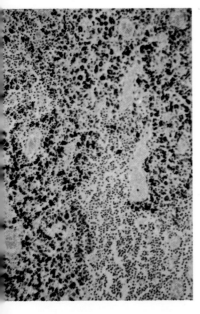
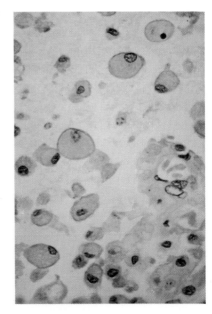
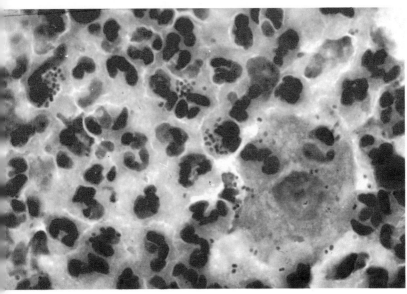

INFLAMMATION: ACUTE

Irrespective of the cause, inflammation occurs whenever cells die or are injured provided that a blood circulation continues in their vicinity. In simple creatures like starfish larvae, with no vascular system, inflammation consists of an accumulation of phagocytes. Development of the vascular system, particularly in homoiotherms, has caused this basically simple process to become exceedingly complex.

An inflamed skin, for example, is hot, red, swollen and painful and one is disinclined to move it. These are the cardinal features of inflammation and most can be explained in terms of the microscopic findings.

The first event, in tissue injury is transient arteriolar constriction followed rapidly by conspicuous and prolonged vasodilatation mainly of capillaries and venules. This is mediated first by histamine from damaged mast cells, later by a variety of vasoactive polypeptides that come from plasma, damaged cells and platelets. These dilated vessels may have such a sluggish flow that the blood clots within them (thrombosis *q.v.*).

In those vessels that have not thrombosed, leucocytes move to the peripheral plasmatic zone, stick to the endothelial surface and migrate between the endothelial cells leaving the vessels and entering the inflamed connective tissues. Polypeptides of 8 to 14 chain length may aid in attracting leucocytes out of vessels and promoting increased permeability.

Plasma and red cells also exude from the dilated vessels and the resultant fluid and cells that appear in the connective tissues is called an inflammatory exudate. If the exudate is caused by bacterial action the organisms may continue to proliferate. Many of the phagocytes and the tissue cells may be killed by the bacterial toxins and the resultant necrotic material is called pus. Pus bordered by inflammatory reaction is called an abscess. It may be acute, as we have described here, or it may last much longer when it is said to be a chronic abscess.

An abscess in a hair follicle is called a boil. It bursts because the tension inside it stretches the overlying epidermis that becomes ischaemic and dies. The boil then bursts, pus is released, and healing begins. The healing phase is called chronic inflammation and comes on about 48 hours after the start of an uncomplicated acute inflammatory response.

Fig. 156. Mast cells in mesenteric connective tissue. They are filled with metachromatic granules that stain purple (Toluidine blue x 350)

Fig. 157. Mast cells stained to show the granules as red (Solachrome cyanin x 880)

Fig. 158. Acute inflammatory exudation in an alveolus. Note dilated capillaries and erythrocytes and leucocytes in the alveolar lumen (H and E x 350)

Fig. 159. High power view of an acute inflammatory exudate showing fibrin (red) and polymorphonuclear leucocytes (H and E x 550)

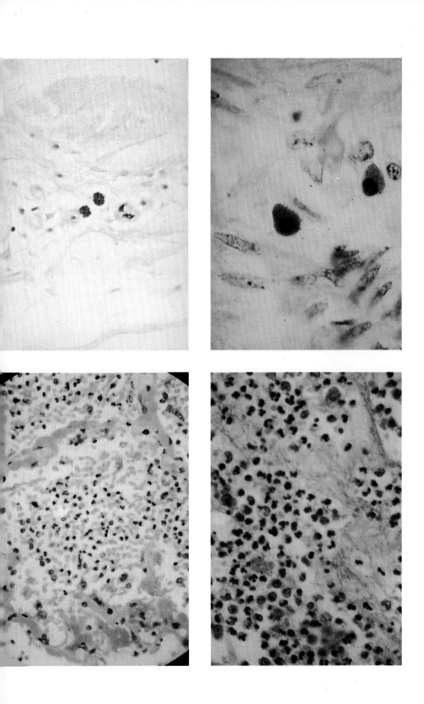

INFLAMMATION
(ACUTE)

Fig. 160. Margination of polymorphonuclear neutrophil leucocytes in a venule in an inflamed tissue. Many leucocytes have left the vessel and fill the surrounding tissue (H and E x 350)

Fig. 161. Thrombosis in a venule in the wall of an inflamed vermiform appendix (H and E x 90)

Fig. 162. A loculated collection of pus (pustule) in the superficial epidermis. An early stage of acute cutaneous infection (H and E x 310)

Fig. 163. Acute fibrinous pleurisy. Note the thin, red film of surface fibrin, leucocytes and dilated vessels in the pleural connective tissue. The black material is carbon in subpleural lymphatics (H and E x 90)

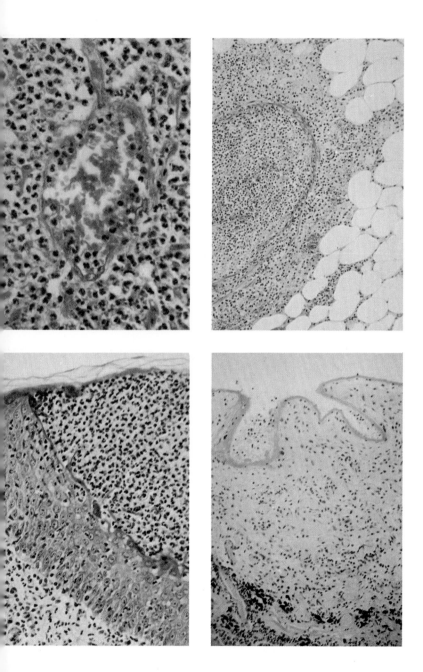

Fig. 164. Fibrinous peri-
carditis. Compare with the
fibrinous pleurisy (H and
E x 35)

Fig. 165. A higher power
view of fibrinous pericar-
ditis (H and E x 220)

Fig. 166. The wall of an
abscess. The inner part (at
the top) consists of polymorphonuclear leucocytes.
The rest of the wall is made
of granulation tissue (*q.v.*)
(H and E x 90)

Fig. 167. Threads of fibrin
in an alveolus. This is early
acute inflammation in lobar
pneumonia. (Mallory's
phosphotungstic acid hae-
matoxylin x 350)

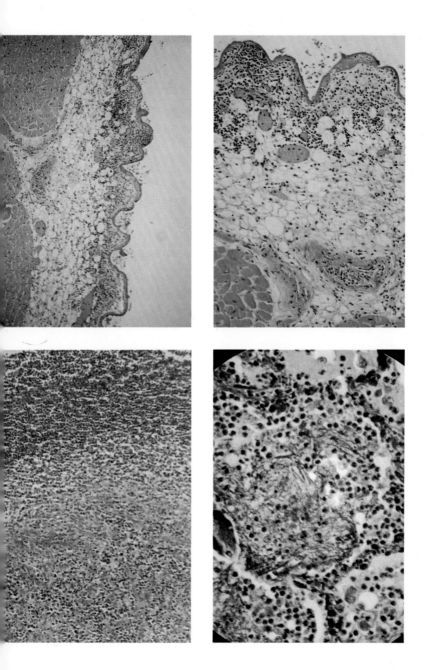

INFLAMMATION: CHRONIC

At about 48 hours after the inflammatory response has started fibroblasts appear; they are derived from fixed mesenchymal cells and they start to elaborate collagen. Young collagen is very like reticulin ($2 \cdot 7$ nm periodicity); it matures to adult collagen later ($6 \cdot 4$ nm). If tension is applied to the healing area the fibroblasts align in parallel rows; if the tension is intermittent then elastic tissue forms as well as collagen. Vascularisation of the newly formed tissue is achieved by solid cords of endothelial cells that bud from adjacent capillaries, later becoming canalised and rejoining the parent vessel by forming a capillary loop.

A special situation exists in the central nervous system where chronic inflammation is accompanied by a proliferation of the glial cells that normally are found there. Polymorphonuclear leucocytes are the principle phagocytes in the acute phase but microglia appear in the chronic phase. These are usually inconspicuous cells with thin flat nuclei; when they devour damaged brain tissue they fill with droplets of lipoid and are called Gitterzellen or compound granular corpuscles.

Chronic lesions in the central nervous system do have collagen and fibroblasts in them because fibroblasts can get into the CNS from the connective sheaths of penetrating blood vessels. The principle cell, however, in chronic processes in the CNS is the astrocyte: a plump cell with a slightly eccentric nucleus. This is a glial cell and produces lots of glial fibres that are concerned with repair processes in the brain and spinal cord.

Fig. 168. Rows of fibro-blasts in a healing wound. Note the polymorpho-nuclear leucocytes, some of which are necrotic (H and E x 350)

Fig. 169. Abundant eosinophil leucocytes in early chronic inflammation. These cells often denote some kind of hypersensitivity and are often seen in worm infestations (H and E x 350)

Fig. 170. Astrocytes in chronic inflammation in the brain. Note the eccentric nuclei and the ragged cyto-plasm (H and E x 350)

Fig. 171. Impregnation of astrocytes with gold, show-ing the star-like processes and the foot-processes attached to a blood vessel (Cajal's gold sublimate x 350)

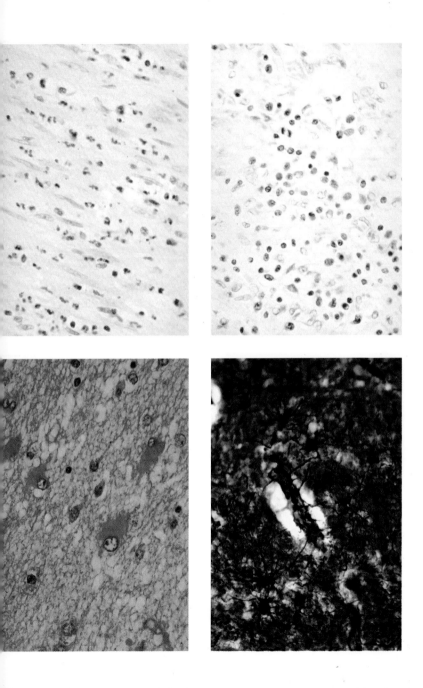

INFLAMMATION: CHRONIC

Granulation Tissue

A boil that has burst on to the skin surface produces a break in the epidermal surface; any such break in an epithelial surface is called an ulcer. Viewed with a hand lens the base of the ulcer consists of tiny red pin points, these are the newly formed capillary loops and have led to the name granulation tissue being applied to it.

Granulation tissue then is composed of:—

(1) Dilated and thrombosed vessels;
(2) Newly formed capillaries;
(3) Inflammatory exudate containing "acute" inflammatory cells *e.g.* polymorphonuclear leucocytes and chronic inflammatory cells such as fibroblasts, macrophages, lymphocytes and later, as a result of the antigenic stimulus from the inflamed area, plasma cells. Quite often binucleate plasma cells are found in chronic inflammatory processes together with circular, amorphous pink Russell bodies that are probably related to antibody formation.

Fig. 172. Fibroblasts, new capillaries and polymorphonuclear leucocytes in a healing wound (H and E x 350)

Fig. 173. Sheaves of fibroblasts in a healing wound (H and E x 90)

Fig. 174. Higher power view of fibroblasts (H and E x 220)

Fig. 175. Fibroblasts to show nuclear detail. Note the conspicuous nucleolus (H and E x 350)

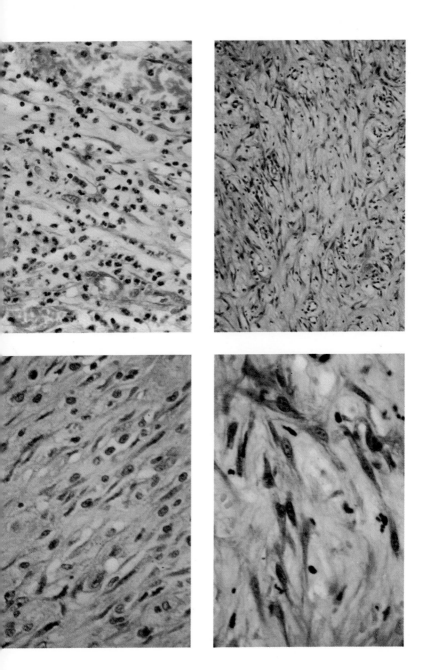

INFLAMMATION
(CHRONIC)

Fig. 176. Fibrin on the surface and coarser, more eosinophilic fibrinoid material in an ulcer (H and E x 220)

Fig. 177. An ulcer in the vermiform appendix: this is an early stage of acute appendicitis. The epithelial surface is above left; the ulcer is below left. Note the granulation tissue in the base of the ulcer (H and E x 90)

Fig. 178. A cutaneous ulcer. The normal epidermis is on the left (H and E x 90)

Fig. 179. A chronic peptic ulcer. The surface is composed of necrotic debris (H and E x 90)

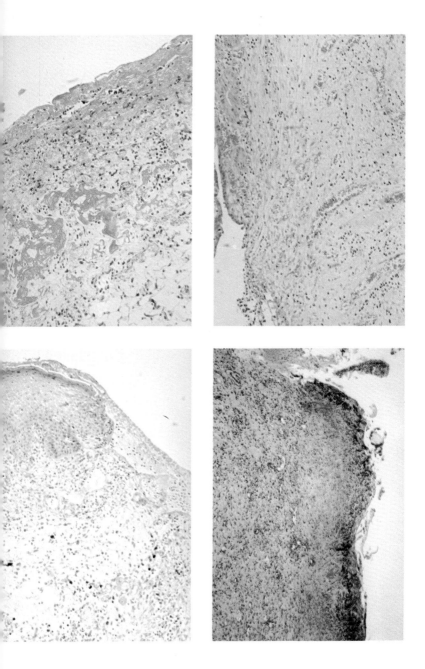

Fig. 180. A polypoid nodule of granulation tissue. These polyps (*q.v.*) are commonly seen on the cervix uteri and in the middle ear (H and E x 90)

Fig. 181. A higher power view of a granulomatous polyp showing new capillaries, inflammatory cells and pink oedema fluid (H and E x 220)

Fig. 182. New capillaries mingled with chronic inflammatory cells and a few polymorphonuclear leucocytes in granulation tissue (H and E x 350)

Fig. 183. Russell bodies, plasma cells, fibroblasts and haemosiderin pigment in granulation tissue (H and E x 350)

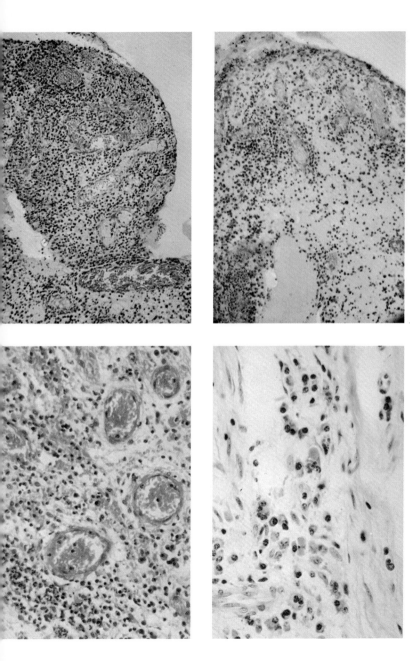

Fig. 184. Newly formed capillaries with plump endothelial cells in a healing wound (H and E x 220)

Fig. 185. Chronic inflammatory reaction (*above*) at the edge of a pulmonary infarct (*below*) (H and E x90)

Fig. 186. Chronic inflammatory infiltrate around a bronchiole from a child with recurrent lung infections (H and E x 90)

Fig. 187. Cirrhosis of the liver. A nodule of surviving liver cells surrounded by fibrous tissue, chronic inflammatory cells and several regenerated bile ductules (H and E x 90)

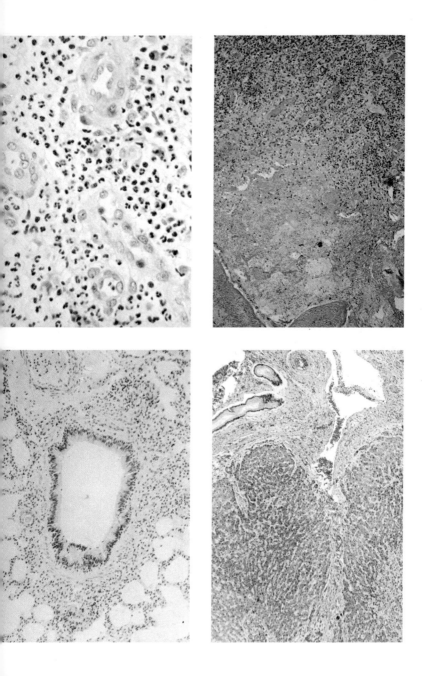

INFLAMMATION: CHRONIC

Granuloma

We have already said that necrosis can be modified by the causative agent; the same applies to inflammation so that it is sometimes possible, by looking at a section of an inflammatory process, to speculate upon what might be the cause of it.

Viral infections tend to produce a mononuclear response of macrophages and lymphoid cells rather than polymorphonuclear cells. Some bacteria produce a lot of pus and are said to be pyogenic (*e.g. Staphylococcus* and *Streptococcus*). Other bacteria like the *Salmonella typhi* produce a chronic inflammatory response and macrophages form the main component of the lesion.

Many organisms, particularly certain bacteria, fungi and metazoa cause a nodular inflammatory response. The cells concerned are tightly packed and clearly circumscribed to form a lesion that is called a *granuloma*. It is not easy to define a granuloma because is consists of a variety of different chronic inflammatory cells that appear in widely differing proportions in different diseases. The cells that are found in granulomas are :—

(1) *Macrophages;*
(2) *Lymphocytes;*
(3) *Plasma cells;*
(4) *Fibroblasts forming collagen;*
(5) *Giant cells.*

As we have said the proportions of these components vary greatly and this variation may provide diagnostic histological criteria for the recognition of the cause of the granuloma. Taking each component of the granuloma in turn :—

Macrophages may constitute the sole feature of the granuloma in leprosy. Here the nodule, from the skin, consists solely of spindle-shaped cells packed with intracellular acid alcohol fast bacilli. Such closely packed macrophages come to resemble columnar epithelial cells and are sometimes called epithelioid cells *(q.v.)*.

Lymphocytes are often present in granulomas usually round the edge. Occasionally they form the bulk of the lesion as in the nodules in joints and lung in rheumatoid disease and in myco-plasmal infections that we have already studied. In some of the auto-allergic diseases, like Hashimoto's disease *(q.v.)* the thyroid is almost entirely replaced by lymphoid tissue giving rise to the so-called "struma lymphomatosa".

Plasma cells are lymphoid cells with a rich endoplasmic reticu-lum that have differentiated to the sole task of antibody produc-tion. Their cytological features have already been described. They preponderate in granulomas of the upper respiratory tract (middle ear infections, pharynx and tonsil), so much so that there is sometimes doubt whether they are neoplastic or granulomatous conditions. Plasma cells abound in chronic diseases such as syphilis ; binucleate plasma cells and Russell bodies are frequently present too.

Fibroblasts may form the bulk of fungal granulomas and granulomas that form around inert foreign particles such as silicon dioxide in the lung. Seaweed extracts such as carrageenin are used experimentally to produce fibroblastic proliferations.

Fig. 188. Chronic inflammatory cells in thickened alveolar walls in the lung; a feature of some virus infections (H and E x 350)

Fig. 189. A cluster of pale staining macrophages in a mesenteric lymph node from a case of typhoid fever (H and E x 350)

Fig. 190. Two foci of caseous necrosis in a tuberculous lymph node (H and E x 90)

Fig. 191. Circumscribed pulmonary nodules of chronic inflammatory cells and fibroblasts around central fragments of schistosomal larvae (H and E x 90)

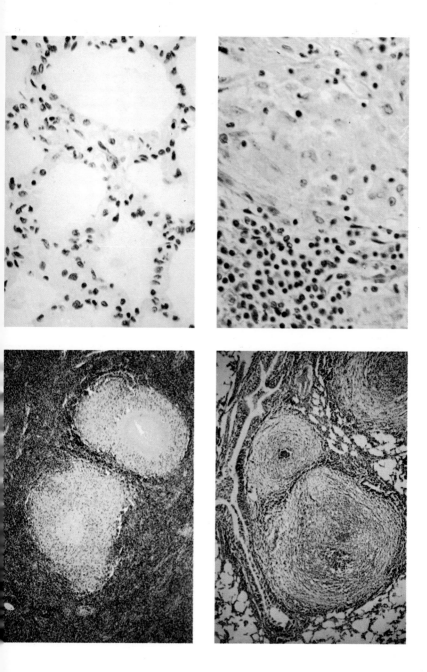

Fig. 192. Fronds of synovium many of which are cut transversely showing foci of lymphocytes and plasma cells. From a case of rheumatoid arthritis (H and E x 35)

Fig. 193. Lung showing a fibrous silicotic nodule (*above*). The black material is a mixture of silica and coal dust (H and E x 90)

Fig. 194. Thyroid acini *(above)*; most of the thyroid gland has been replaced by lymphoid cells (Hashimoto's disease) (H and E x 220)

Fig. 195. Thyroid (Hashimoto's disease) showing compressed, angular thyroid cells (Askanazy cells) above (H and E x 220)

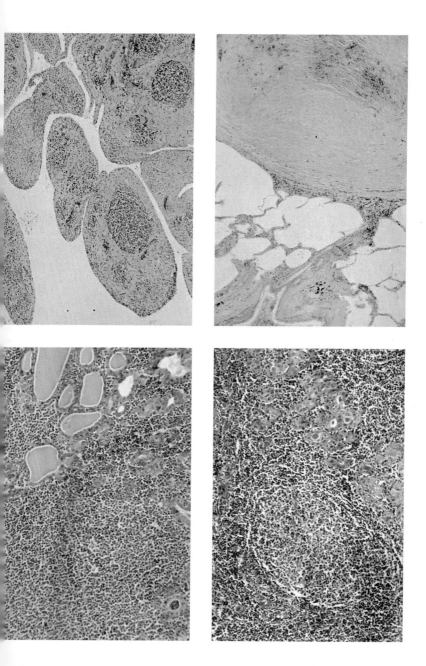

INFLAMMATION: CHRONIC

Giant Cells

Giant cells appear in many kinds of granuloma. Originally it was thought that specific sorts of giant cells were associated with particular diseases. The more one looks at them the less likely does this seem to be true. Giant cells are either formed by the fusion of macrophages or by the division of macrophage nuclei without cytoplasmic cleavage; the former seems to be more likely. The simplest sort of giant cell forms around foreign body particles such as catgut, wood, etc. The foreign particle that elicits the reaction can often be seen in an ordinary H and E preparation viewed in visible light. Occasionally one has to resort to the use of polarised light. Here use is made of the ability of the crystalline foreign object to deflect the parallel rays of polarised light so that the object shows brightly against a black ground. Any object, solid or liquid, that has an orderly arrangement of molecules in it is able to deflect polarised light and is said to be anisotropic or birefringent.

Fig. 196. A giant cell related to a starch grain in the lung of a drug addict who had injected herself with powdered barbiturate tablets (H and E x 350)

Fig. 197. Starch grain in the lung seen by polarised light. Note that crystalline material in the mountant is also birefringent (H and E x 220)

Fig. 198. A cluster of giant cells around a foreign body (needle fragment) in the dermis (H and E x 220)

Fig. 199. Giant cells, fibroblasts and a few lymphocytes in a fungal granuloma (H and E x 220)

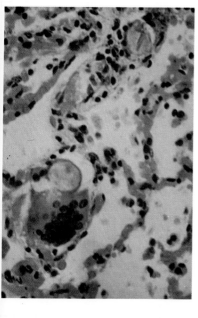
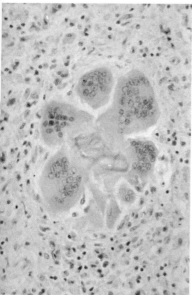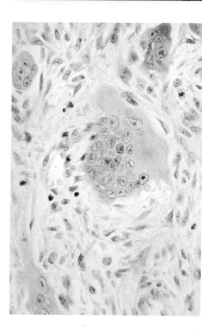

Fig. 200. Pieces of catgut in an old surgical scar. Sometimes this material elicits a giant-cell reaction (McFarlane's modification of Mallory's trichrome x 220)

Fig. 201. A hair shaft growing in the dermis; this can act as a foreign body and elicit a giant cell reaction (H and E x 90)

Fig. 202. Giant cells containing haemosiderin in an old subcutaneous haemorrhage (H and E x 350)

Fig. 203. Giant cells at the edge of necrotic tissue in a benign neoplasm (*q.v.*) of the skin (H and E x 220)

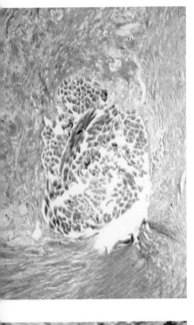
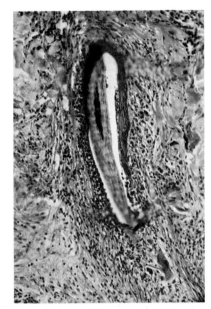
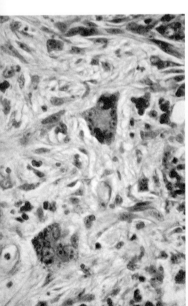
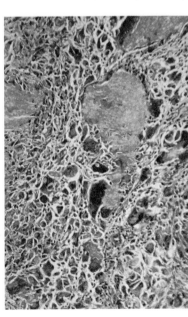

Fig. 204. Cholesterol clefts (the lipoid has dissolved in processing) calcium above.
Cholesterol often initiates a giant cell response (H and E x 90)

Fig. 205. Giant cells and other chronic inflammatory cells in necrotic fatty tissue. One giant cell contains a globule of fat (H and E x 90)

Fig. 206. A giant celled granuloma in the myocardium. This is giant celled myocarditis and the cause is obscure (H and E x 90)

Fig. 207. Lipoid pneumonia. Spaces that contained fat bordered by dense fibrous tissue and occasional giant cells. Caused by the inhalation of oil into the lungs (H and E x·35)

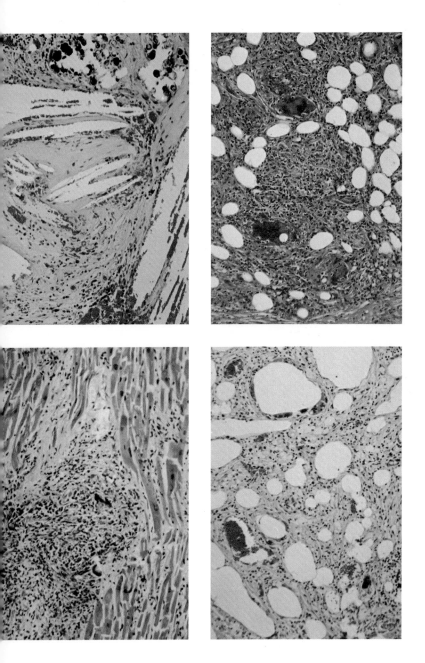

INFLAMMATION: CHRONIC

Giant Cells

Living foreign agents as well as inert foreign matter cause giant cells to appear. Tuberculosis is a good example where the cells are large and have many nuclei scattered around the periphery of the cell; these are called Langhan's giant cells. Giant cells are often seen in fungal infections, particularly those fungi that penetrate into the deep tissues rather than those that colonise the surface (*e.g.* athlete's foot). Some of the viruses encourage giant cells to form; one group known as respiratory syncytial viruses (RSV) are notable in this respect for they cause giant cells to form in tissue cultures infected by them; another is measles virus. At the other end of the parasitic scale bits of metazoan parasites induce giant cell formation; here they are acting more as foreign bodies.

Fig. 208. So-called Langhan's giant cell in a tuberculous follicle in the liver (H and E x 90)

Fig. 209. Giant cell in a lymphoid follicle from a cervical lymph node. This is the Warthin-Finkeldey giant cell of measles (H and E x 350)

Fig. 210. Bloated · pale giant cells, some of which are necrotic, derived from epidermal cells in herpes virus infection (H and E x 350)

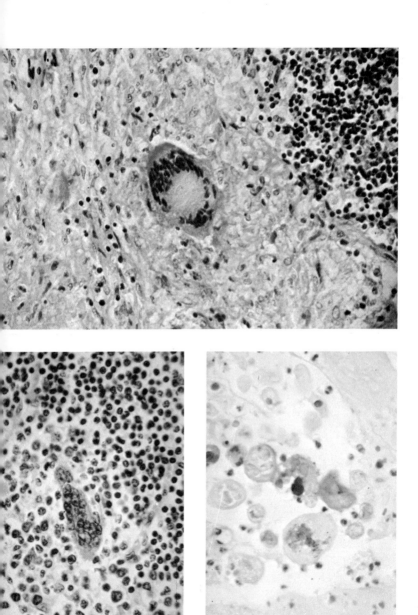

Fig. 211. Giant celled arteritis showing a band of pink necrosis in the arterial wall (H and E x 90)

Fig. 212. Giant celled arteritis. An artefactual cleft has formed in the wall; there are giant cells along both edges of the cleft. Note the internal elastic lamella (H and E x 90)

Fig. 213. Giant celled arteritis showing fragments of the original internal elastica near the artefactual cleft. The inner black lamellae are newly formed. The lumen is filled with organised thrombus (q.v.) that is canalised (q.v.) (Hart's modification of Weigert's elastic stain x 90)

Fig. 214. The same artery showing the giant cell more clearly. Giant celled arteritis may be an autoallergic reaction (q.v.) to elastin. (Mallory's phosphotungstic acid haematoxylin x 90)

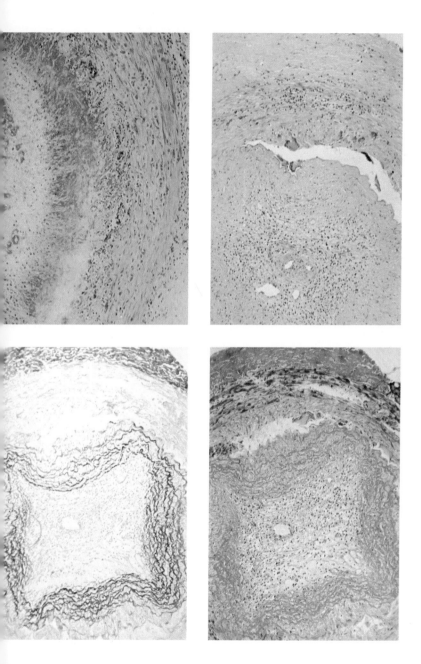

INFLAMMATION: CHRONIC

Giant Cells

The classical granuloma is that seen in tuberculosis where there is central necrosis and more peripheral epithelioid cells, giant cells and lymphocytes. Suitable staining methods (Ziehl Neelsen) demonstrate the organism as slightly curved red rods sometimes finely beaded along their length and arranged in clumps.

Generally speaking, the granuloma suggests to the histologist that some sort of hypersensitivity mechanism is operative. This is so in tuberculosis snd many other disorders such as syphilis, various sorts of arteritis, and so on.

One of the most mysterious granulomatous diseases is sarcoidosis (literally fleshy disease) where many parts of the reticuloendothelial system are enlarged (lymph nodes, spleen, liver) and contain granulomas that are also present in other tissues such as skin, bone, eye, lungs, heart, etc.

The cause of sarcoidosis is obscure, though some think that inhalation of pine pollen is a factor. Giant cells are a conspicuous feature of the granulomas of this disease and contain a variety of structures. The granulomas are very like those of tuberculosis but there is no central necrosis (caseation). Giant cells may contain globular bodies, asteroid bodies and Schaumann bodies. None of these is specific for giant cells of sarcoidosis. In fact, the sarcoid granuloma is not specific for the recognition of sarcoidosis, such granulomas may be present in a variety of conditions:

(1) Around insect bites in the skin;
(2) In lymph nodes draining sites of carcinoma (*q.v.*);
(3) In relation to blood shed into the tissues;
(4) In the lungs after inhalation of beryllium dust;
(5) In farmer's lung due to the inhalation of fungus *Thermospora* from mouldy hay.

Granulomas are often found in the gut wall, notably in ileum, colon and to a lesser extent stomach. They are associated with a chronic, localised thickening of the gut caused by diffuse chronic inflammation of the wall. This is called regional ileitis, regional colitis or Crohn's disease. The cause is obscure and granulomas appear late in the disease; again they may be due to repeated sensitisation of the injured gut wall by foreign material penetrating from the lumen of the gut.

GIANT CELLS
(SARCOIDOSIS)

Fig. 215. Lymph node largely replaced by sarcoid granulomas (H and E x 35)

Fig. 216. A higher power view of sarcoid granulomas showing giant cells embedded in macrophages but no caseation as in tuberculosis (H and E x 90)

Fig. 217. Sarcoid granuloma in the wall of the colon in regional colitis (Crohn's disease) (H and E x 35)

Fig. 218. An asteroid body in a giant cell from a sarcoid granuloma (H and E x 350)

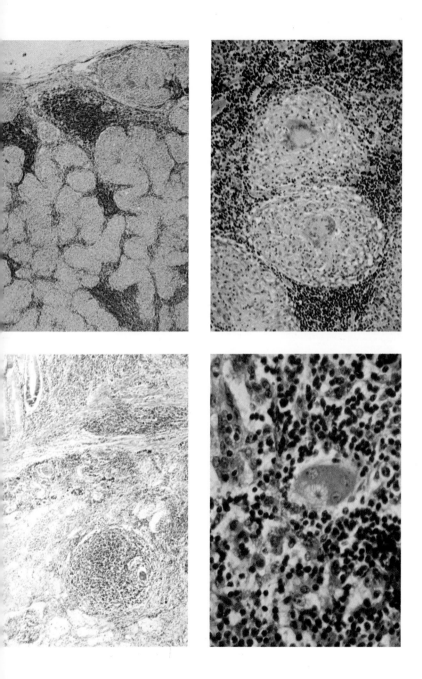

GIANT CELLS
(SARCOIDOSIS)

Fig. 219. Sarcoidosis: an asteroid body in the giant cell (left) and globular bodies in the giant cell to the right of it (H and E x 350)

Fig. 220. Globular bodies in a giant cell associated with a foreign body reaction to lipoid (H and E x 220)

Fig. 221. A Schaumann (conchoidal) body on the left has a blue, faintly laminated appearance; a giant cell on the right (H and E x 500)

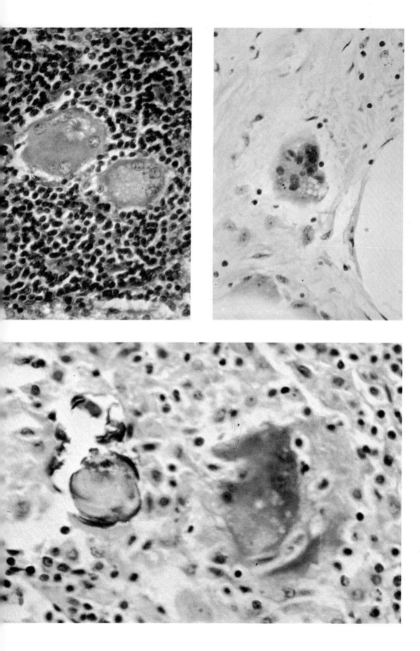

REPAIR AND REGENERATION

Repair of a damaged tissue follows, or rather may follow, the acute inflammatory process if the aggravating cause is eliminated or suppressed. We have already considered chronic inflammation and this is part of the repair process. Broadly repair consists of :—

(1) *Removal* of necrotic debris (phagocytosis).
(2) *Replacement* of dead tissue either by collagen (repair by scarring) or by the appearance of new cells of the tissue to replace the damaged ones (regeneration).

Repair by scarring commonly occurs when highly specialised structures are destroyed. For example, a deep cut in the scalp heals by scarring; this leaves a bald patch because the specialised hair follicles fail to regenerate in the scar. The less specialised epidermis is however capable of regeneration and grows over the surface of the scar thus producing healing of the wound. Mitoses are often very frequent in such regenerating epidermis and it is important not to confuse this active normal tissue with a neoplasm (*q.v.*).

Liver readily regenerates after pieces have been excised or destroyed in some other way. Again, abundant mitoses in the liver cells may give a false impression of neoplasia.

Some structures like axons and skeletal muscle cells are quite capable of regeneration provided the neurilemmal and sarcolemmal tubules persist in the damaged tissue. If an axon is crushed but the neurone is intact then a new axon grows into the neurilemmal tube distal to the crushing. It follows that axonal regeneration does not occur in the central nervous system where there are no such neurilemmal structures. Crushed skeletal muscle behaves in the same way; new myoblasts and myofilaments appear from swollen sarcolemmal nuclei and these fill the sarcolemmal tube. If the sarcolemma is transected then a knot of newly formed myoblasts, with nowhere to go, forms yet another kind of giant cell; a muscle giant cell.

Factors concerned in regeneration are poorly understood.

REPAIR AND REGENERATION

Fig. 222. A pink, collagenous scar in the skin. There are sweat glands at the edge of the scar and compressed vessels at the edge (H and E x 90)

Fig. 223. Several mitoses in regenerating liver cells (H and E x 220)

Fig. 224. Regenerating skeletal muscle (*above*) showing newly formed myofibrils in the sarcolemmal tube. Necrotic, eosinophilic muscle below (H and E x 220)

Fig. 225. Chains of enlarged sarcolemmal nuclei (*above*) in regenerating muscle from an area of haemorrhage; note the haemosiderin pigment

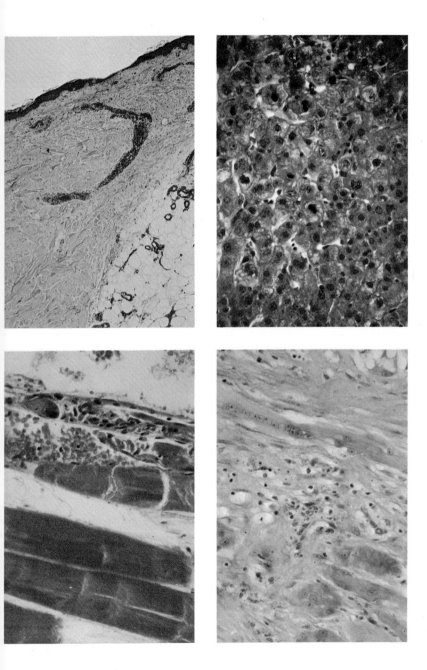

Patterns of Disease

INFECTION

INFECTIONS may remain confined to a particular organ in which they arise or they may spread widely to produce septicaemia and death: lung infections provide a diversity of reactions due to differing properties of the agents that cause them.

Bacterial infections may be pyogenic or not, as we have seen. Many bacteria that gain entry to the lung, when the epithelial barriers are destroyed by cold, age, smoke, and poisons, cause purulent infiltrations in the lung. They occur in bronchioles and in the adjacent alveoli usually in the dependent lower lobes of the lungs. This is called bronchopneumonia and is often preceded by bronchitis (bronchial and bronchiolar inflammation).

Bronchopneumonia is, then, a patchy process scattered throughout the lower lobes. Adjacent alveoli may be collapsed because the respiratory bronchiole is blocked by pus from the bronchopneumonic area. Other alveoli may be compensatorily dilated (so-called emphysema). Appearances in bronchopneumonia vary according to the nature of the organism and its virulence. Staphylococci may cause haemorrhagic pneumonia where much blood is present in alveoli; this is an effect of the α toxin. Occasionally if the virulence of the organism is high the bronchopneumonic areas may coalesce so that the whole lobe is involved (confluent bronchopneumonia) and furthermore intense necrosis, in such a lobe, may lead to abscess formation.

Lobar pneumonia is a different disease. It is usually caused by a pneumococcus and is peculiar in that the whole lobe or lobule of the lung is uniformly involved right from the start of the process.

The disease progresses in stages over a period of about eight days after which the patient may recover completely and dramatically. Early on the changes in the alveoli are those of acute inflammation: the alveolar exudate contains fibrin, erythrocytes and abundant pneumococci. Later the character of the exudate changes, becoming more purulent and the pneumococci disappear. Later still, macrophages appear to clear away the intra-alveolar debris and the lung returns to normal. An exudate of fibrin always appears on the pleural surface, in lobar pneumonia, because the whole lobe is uniformly involved. This uniform involvement is one of the mysteries of lobar pneumonia and may be due to a hypersensitivity mechanism *(q.v.)*.

Fig. 226. Squamous metaplasia of bronchial epithelium. The basement mem-
brane is well illustrated
(Mallory's phosphotungstic
acid haematoxylin x 350)

Fig. 227. Excessive
mucous-gland activity often
associated with squamous
metaplasia in chronic
bronchitis (Alcian blue x
90)

Fig. 228. Purulent bronchitis showing pus in the
bronchiole (*above*), part of
the intact epithelium and
dilated capillaries in the
bronchial wall (H and E x
90)

Fig. 229. Broncho-
pneumonia showing
leucocytes in a bronchiole
and leucocytes in some of
the adjacent alveoli. The
process is patchy and
centred upon the bron-
chiole (H and E x 35)

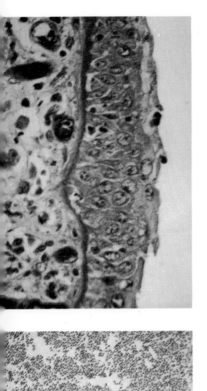
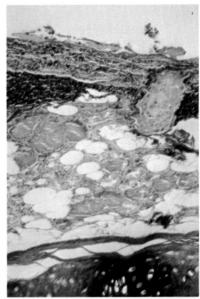
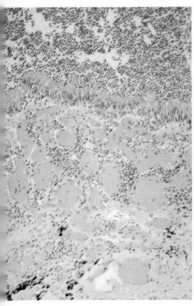
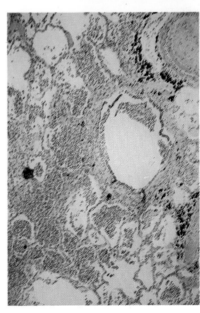

Fig. 230. Acute haemorrhagic staphylococcal pneumonia showing dark areas of consolidation

Fig. 231. A section of acute haemorrhagic pneumonia showing much blood in alveoli (H and E x 44)

Fig. 232. Bronchopneumonia showing the patchy nature of the process (H and E x 35)

Fig. 233. Lobar pneumonia; note the uniform nature of the process. Alveoli contain polymorphonuclear neutrophil leucocytes (H and E x 90)

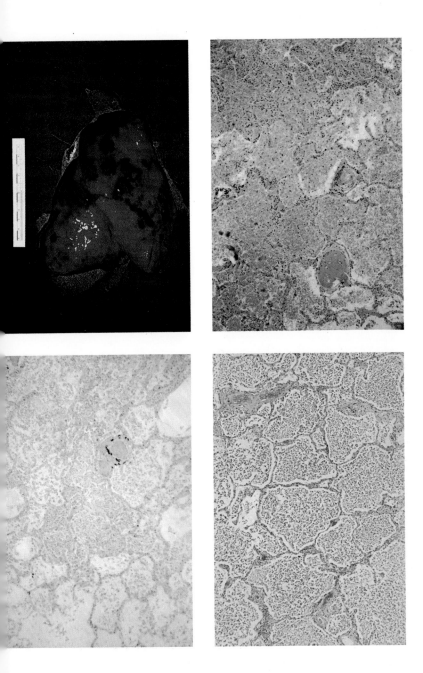

PATTERNS OF DISEASE

Infection

A wide variety of bacteria may cause acute purulent bronchitis and bronchopneumonia; these are acute infections that either kill the patient or are resolved in a matter of days. More chronic, long standing disorders of the lung are caused by organisms such as fungi and mycobacteria; the best known of these is tuberculosis. In children this leads to caseation in the lung (Ghon focus) and in the draining lymph node; the two lesions are called the primary complex. In the adult the lung lesion is better confined by a fibrous capsule and spread to the local lymph node does not occur. Some think that this is due to the protective hypersensitivity conferred by the primary infection of childhood.

If either primary (childhood) or secondary (adult) lesions rupture into a blood vessel then tuberculous material is spread over the body giving rise to small tuberculous granulomas in many organs (kidney, liver, spleen, adrenals, meninges). This is called miliary tuberculosis and was a uniformly fatal disorder before the advent of tuberculostatic drugs.

Miliary tuberculosis is an example of septicaemic spread of the *Myco. tuberculosis* from a local lesion in the lung or from local lesions elsewhere in the body.

Fig. 234. Kidney showing caseous, tuberculous necrosis of the pelvis (*below*) and compressed cortex (*above*) (H and E x 35)

Fig. 235. Spleen miliary tuberculosis; one tuberculous follicle adjacent to several Malphighian bodies (H and E x 35)

Fig. 236. Lung miliary tuberculosis (H and E x 35)

Fig. 237. Liver showing one tuberculous follicle at the edge of the section. From a case of miliary tuberculosis (H and E x 35)

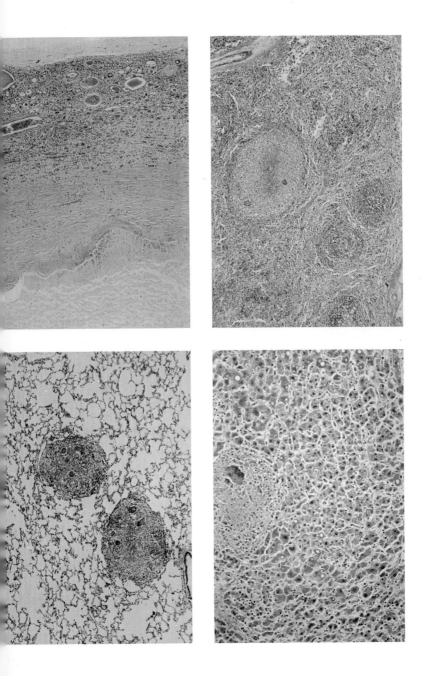

PATTERNS OF DISEASE

Trauma

THERE IS a steady increase in the incidence of traumatic injury on the roads of this country and also as a result of violence in modern society. A study of traumatic lesions is important, particularly to the forensic pathologist, for it often enables the cause and time of the injury to be determined.

The presence of an inflammatory reaction at the edges of a wound obviously indicate that it was sustained before death. The demonstration of haemosiderin in a bruise indicates that the bruise is at least forty-eight hours old, for haemosiderin takes that time to form.

Heat coagulation of tissue at the edge of a wound can be spotted microscopically; if there is blackening of the wound as well this suggests that a cartridge has been discharged at close range as in suicidal shooting, and enables the nature of the missile to be suspected.

By the application of a general knowledge of the processes of inflammation it is possible to determine the age of a wound fairly accurately. This is an important issue in forensic pathology. For example, the recognition of the battered child syndrome, where children are repeatedly beaten and ultimately die, may rest upon the determination of wounds of various ages on and within the body.

TRAUMA

Fig. 238. Extensive recent bruising of subcutaneous tissue over the upper thoracic region caused by a kick from an assailant. Incision is needed to show the extent of the bruise

Fig. 239: Section of a recent bruise. It is not spectacular, consisting only of red blood cells in the adipose tissue (H and E x 90)

Fig. 240. One haemosiderin containing macrophage indicates that the blood pigment was liberated some two days before (Perls' x 220)

Fig. 241. Cerebral cortex showing many small, recent haemorrhages following head injury (H and E x 90)

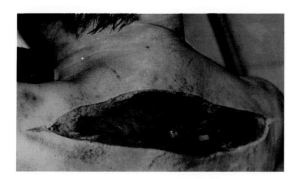

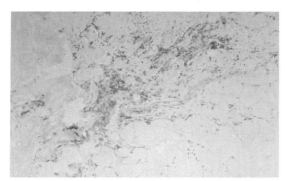

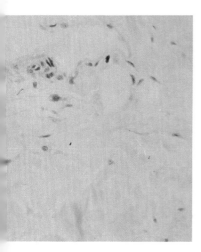

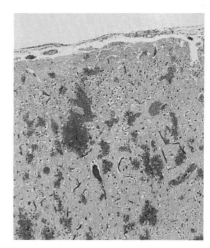

Fig. 242. Pale pink dura mater with organising blood clot on the surface (*above*). This is caused by rotational injury to the skull. (H and E x 220)

Fig. 243. Organising clot on the dura containing haemosiderin (Perls' x 220)

Fig. 244. Suicidal gun-shot wound of head showing blackening of the edge of the wound of entry

Fig. 245. Scorching of epidermis and a superficial deposit of carbon. From the edge of a gun-shot wound (H and E x 90)

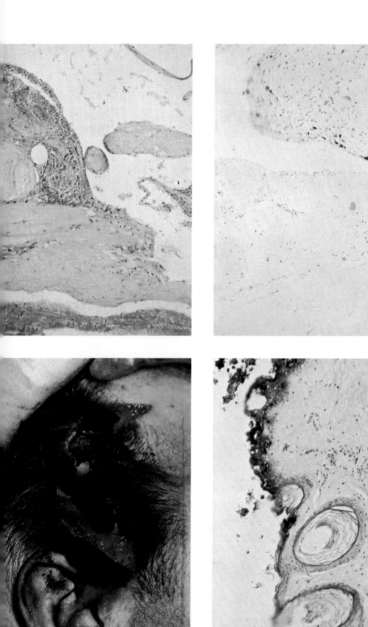

PATTERNS OF DISEASE

Trauma

One of the structures most frequently involved in traumatic injury is bone. The process of healing in bone is similar to healing elsewhere in the body, but is complicated by the appearance of specialised tissues and by the rather redundant use of terminology.

Bone is either compactly arranged as in the cortex of long bones, or loosely arranged as a meshwork as in the marrow space (compact and cancellous bone respectively). In the adult both types are lamellar bone consisting of layers of calcified collagen separating rows of osteocytes in lacunae. Because of its ordered arrangement lamallar bone is birefringent. When new bone forms, as a result of fracture or other disorder, it is not laid down in an orderly way initially. It consists of irregularly arranged osteocytes enclosed in randomly distributed fibres like the arrangement of strands in a ball of string. Such is called woven bone and is not birefringent.

Initially a healing fracture shows a swelling on the bone so-called primary callus. This is composed of fibroblasts, woven bone and variable amounts of cartilage depending on the degree of movement at the fracture site; the greater the mobility of the fracture the greater the amount of cartilage. Secondary callus is complete restoration of bone shape and continuity by the transformation of woven to lamellar bone by the combined action of phagocytic osteoclasts and osteoblasts that produce bone.

Extensive bony injury, *e.g.* multiple fracture of ribs during attempted resuscitation, leads to the liberation of bone marrow into the venous circulation and particles may be seen in sections of pulmonary artery (bone-marrow embolism: *q.v.*).

In old persons, or where extensive fractures occur in the young, fat may be liberated into the venous circulation and block lung capillaries or pass by arteriovenous anastomosis to capillaries in the brain, kidney and heart, causing severe dysfunction there. Similar fat embolism may follow trauma to subcutaneous fat and other fatty tissues independent of that found in the adult bones.

Fig. 246. Lamellar, mature bone (*below*) and woven, new bone (*above*), Note the difference in arrangement of osteocytes (H and E x 90)

Fig. 247. Lamellar bone (*below*) is birefringent. Woven bone (*above*) is only weakly birefringent (H and E, polarised light x 90)

Fig. 248. A high power view of woven bone showing frequent, plump, irregularly arranged osteocytes (H and E x 350)

Fig. 249. A recent fracture showing broken lamellar bone, separated by fibroblasts. Fibrinoid material (*left*) is in the line of the fracture (H and E x 90)

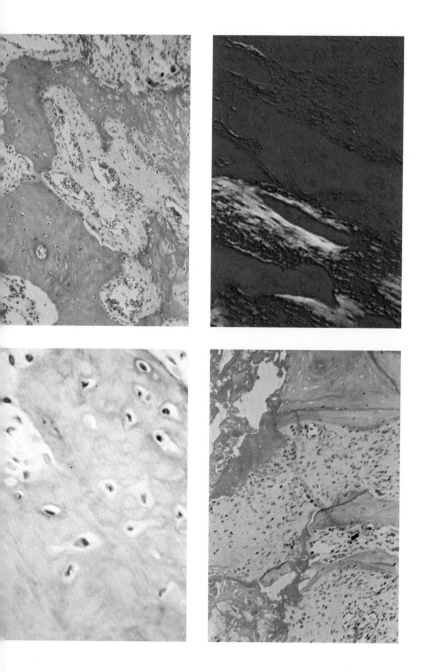

Fig. 250. Primary callus composed of woven bone and cartilage below. Fibrinoid (*left*) adjacent to the fractured mature lamellar bone (H and E x 90)

Fig. 251. Extensive bruising along the pleural aspects of fractured right ribs. This may cause fat and bone marrow embolism

Fig. 252. Bone marrow containing fat cells and haemopoietic cells in a pulmonary artery. From a case of bone marrow embolism (H and E x 90)

Fig. 253. Lung showing extensive plugging of capillaries by red staining fat (Sudan III/IV x 90)

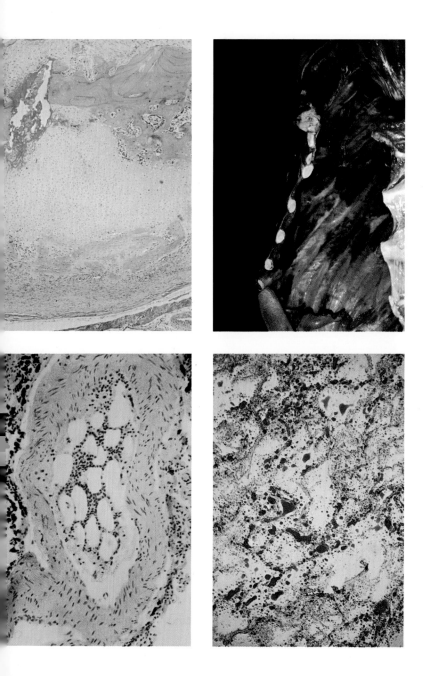

Fig. 254. A higher power view of the lung from a case of fat embolism showing the elongated fat droplets (H and E x 220)

Fig. 255. Renal glomerular capillaries distended with droplets of fat. Processing has dissolved the fat (H and E x 350)

Fig. 256. A thick section of a glomerulus in fat embolism. Note the red globules of fat in glomeruli (Sudan III/IV x 350)

Fig. 257. Brain showing extensive petechial haemorrhages in fat embolism due to extensive capillary blockage by fat

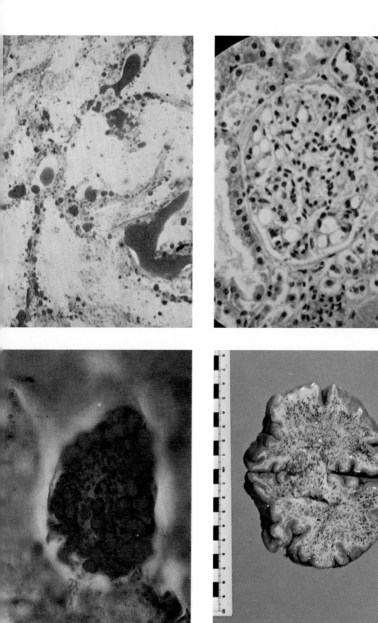

Fig. 258. Haemorhage in brain around a capillary distended by fat (H and E x 124)

Fig. 259. Cerebral capillaries distended by fat droplets (H and E x 124)

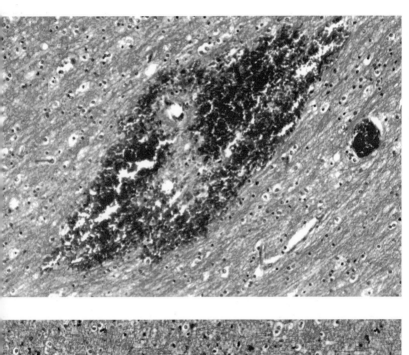
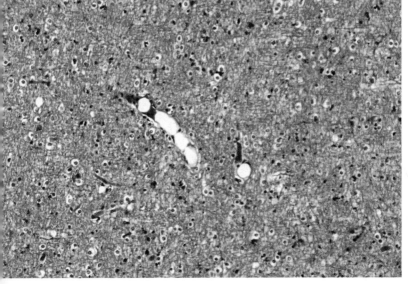

PATTERNS OF DISEASE

Ischaemia

The word literally means "to hold back blood". It is a state where insufficient oxygen gets to the tissues. The causes are vascular obstructions of various kinds:—

(1) *Vascular Disease* leading to narrowing;
(2) *Thrombosis;*
(3) *Mechanical obstruction* such as
    a) Pressure
    b) Ligation
    c) Embolism *i.e.* blockage by particles of material circulating in the blood.

We shall deal, in this chapter, with thrombosis, which is really a sort of mechanical obstruction though worthy of consideration separately, and with other sorts of mechanical blockage of vessels.

Blood clots when it becomes stagnant but this is not thrombosis. A thrombus is an orderly structure made up of layers of platelets, fibrin and red blood cells. The fact that it is layered suggests that it forms as blood flows over the surface, *i.e.* it forms in a living vessel.

Fig. 260. A recent thrombus in a vein showing the layered thrombus (*below*) and the red tail (formed of clot) (*above*) (H and E x 35)

Fig. 261. Details of a thrombus : fibrin (red), platelets (pale mauve), erythrocytes (yellow) (McFarlane's modification of Mallory's trichrome x 90)

Fig. 262. Blue clusters of platelets in a thrombus. Fibrin (red) erythrocytes (yellow) (McFarlane's modification of Mallory's trichrome x 220)

Fig. 263. A vein containing recent thrombus. Vein wall is above; the thrombus separated from it by an artefactual gap (McFarlane's modification of Mallory's trichrome x 90)

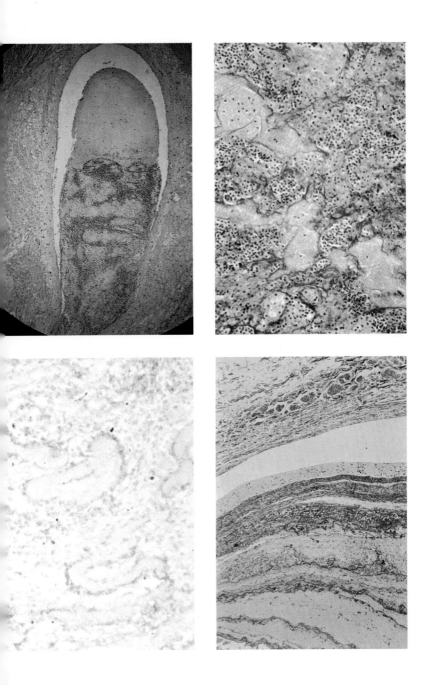

ISCHAEMIA

Thrombosis

Two factors are needed before thrombosis occurs:—
(1) Injury to the vascular endothelium;
(2) Slowing of blood flow in the vessel.
Increase in blood viscosity due either to fluid loss or cellular increase, particularly, of platelets, will further encourage the tendency for thrombi to form.
Several things may happen to thrombi:—
(1) They may be removed by phagocytes or be dissolved by fibrinolysis;
(2) They may propagate so as to block the vessel and its branches;
(3) They may organise by the ingrowth of granulation tissue and the vessel may, ultimately be filled with a fibrous scar;
(4) They may canalise and the vessel lumen is to some extent restored by cracks forming in the thrombus being lined by endothelium or by the complete penetration of the blockage by newly formed capillaries;
(5) Infection of a thrombus may cause it to fragment and liberate particles of infected material into the circulation (pyaemia);
(6) A sterile thrombus, in a vein, may also break loose and impact in a pulmonary artery (pulmonary embolism).

Fig. 264. Cut surface of the right lower lobe of the lung showing recent thrombus in the pulmonary artery

Fig. 265. A post mortem clot taken from the pulmonary artery. Note how it is a perfect cast of the main pulmonary vessels

Fig. 266. Artery filled with organised thrombus; the pink material is collagen. (Hart's modification of Weigert's elastic stain x 90)

Fig. 267. Pale staining atheromatous artery (*q.v.*) (*below*). Organised thrombus (*above*) containing newly formed vascular channels (H and E x 90)

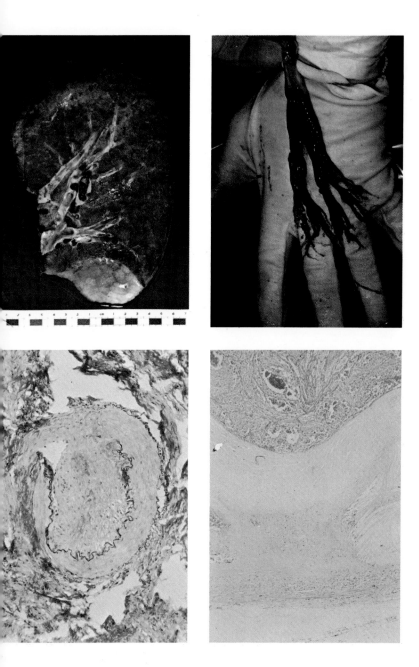

ISCHAEMIA

Embolism and Infarction

Blockage of an artery or a vein may be due to thrombi, air, fat, neoplasm, parasites, foreign bodies, and so on. We have already discussed fat embolism, the effects of air embolism are similar.

The result of vascular blockage is determined by:

(a) The territory that the vessel supplies;
(b) The extent of the collateral circulation;
(c) The state of the collateral vessels; whether they are diseased or not;
(d) The rate of flow of blood through these vessels;
(e) The oxygen carrying power of the blood that is depleted when the haemoglobin level is reduced (anaemia);
(f) The nature and activity of the tissue supplied by the vessel.

When part of an organ becomes ischaemic it dies; the dead tissue shows all the features of necrosis histologically. At the edge of the dead tissue is a zone of acute inflammation from which exudate pours into the necrotic area causing it to become stuffed with exudate and inflammatory cells (infarction). An infarct, then, is an area of ischaemic necrosis. Some infarcts are pale yellow, others deep red. The colour depends on the vascularity of the structure; if there are many leaking vessels at the edge of an infarct, as in the lung, it is red. If the blood supply is radial, as in the kidney then the infarct is pale. Infarcts caused by venous block are consequently often red wherever they occur.

An infarct, like any other inflammatory area, may organise and turn into a sunken scar.

THROMBOSIS AND EMBOLISM

Fig. **268.** Ischaemic necrosis of the hand (gangrene) caused by embolic blockage of the brachial artery

Fig. **269.** A renal artery containing thrombus and cholesterol clefts. This is cholesterol embolism the source is an atheromatous aorta (*q.v.*) (H and E x 90)

Fig. 270. Canalised thrombus in an artery. Note the new vascular channels (H and E x 310)

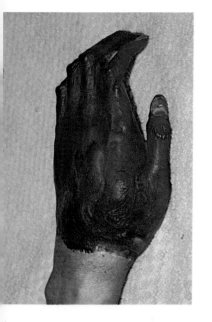
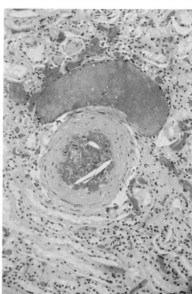
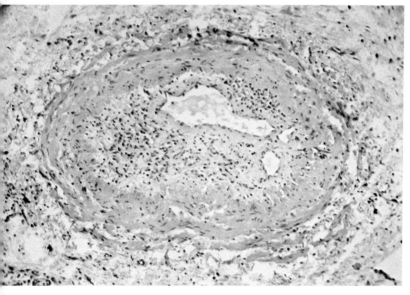

Fig. 271. Splenic infarct showing necrotic tissue above and the adjacent inflammatory reaction (*below*) (H and E x 90)

Fig. 272. Edge of a splenic infarct showing surviving connective tissue cells (H and E x 350)

Fig. 273. Cardiac infarct; dead eosinophilic muscle on the left, inflammatory response on the right (H and E x124)

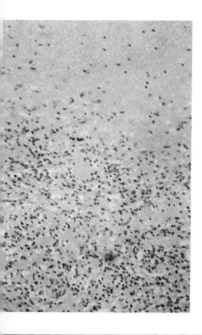

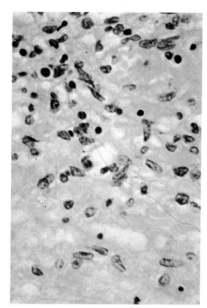

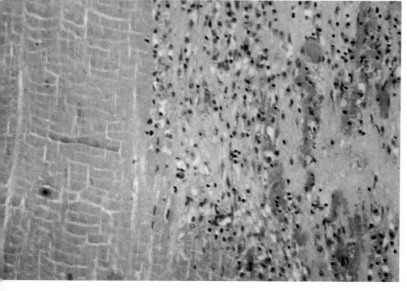

PATTERNS OF DISEASE

Ischaemia

If ischaemia is gradual as may occur with progressive arterio-sclerosis (*q.v.*) in organs such as heart, kidney and brain, then the tissue affected shrinks gradually and is slowly replaced by fibrous tissue.

Ischaemia causes local hypoxia. General hypoxia occurs when oxygen supply to cells is reduced. This is seen in an anaemia when fatty change may occur in a variety of organs such as heart and liver. If the hypoxia persists then the cells die.

Anaemia is due to:
(1) Blood loss;
(2) Red cell lysis;
(3) Inadequate red cell formation.

The histological features in anaemia are not often conspicuous. If lysis is the cause then abundant haemosiderin collects in the liver and spleen. This is also seen in some examples of inadequate red cell formation.

Fig. 274. An ischaemic glomerulus caused by arteriosclerotic narrowing of a renal artery (*q.v.*). The glomerulus is replaced by hyaline collagen (H and E x 220)

Fig. 275. An ischaemic glomerulus staining blue. Early ischaemic changes in the adjacent glomerulus consist of blue, collagenous thickening of the parietal layer of Bowman's capsule (McFarlane's modification of Mallory's trichrome x 90)

Fig. 276. Subcapsular fatty change in the liver commonly due to hypoxia (McFarlane's modification of Mallory's trichrome x 90)

Fig. 277. Clusters of haemosiderin laden macrophages around a splenic arteriole. From a case of haemolytic anaemia (H and E x 350)

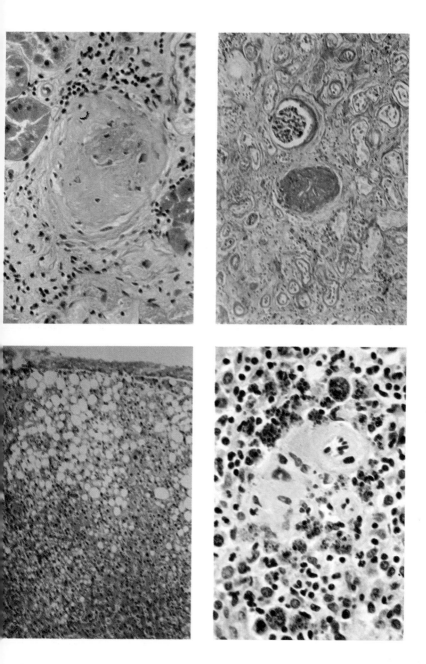

PATTERNS OF DISEASE

Degeneration

This is an unfortunate term implying progressive collapse of the fabric of the body with age. It is true that a variety of events come on with age. The bones become fragile and lose their trabeculae (osteoporosis). The collagen of the dermis fragments and takes up stains for elastic tissue (so called "senile" elastosis); this change occurs on the facial skin and may not necessarily be the result of age but due to prolonged solar exposure. Lipochrome pigment collects in liver, heart and neurones of the aged. Cerebral vessels become encrusted with iron and calcium and the media of thyroid, uterine, ovarian and other vessels tends to calcify.

Probably the most important event that progresses with age is the gradual narrowing of many blood vessels by intimal thickening. This is one form of *arteriosclerosis* which is a generic, non-specific term for several kinds of arterial thickening. Arteriosclerosis comprises:

(1) *Intimal* fibro-elastic and muscular thickening seen in small arteries;
(2) *Atherosclerosis* which starts as an intimal accumulation of lipids, collagen and elastic fibrils and smooth muscle cells. Later the media is affected. It is a disease of large arteries;
(3) *Mönckeberg's sclerosis* which is an unimportant medial calcification of the long arteries of the limbs. It has little effect on the vascular lumen;
(4) *Various sorts* of vasculitis, acute and chronic seen in hypersensitivity disorders (*q.v.*)

Fig. 278. Osteoporosis of vertebrae. Note the thin sparse trabeculae and white disc material that has prolapsed into the vertebral body

Fig. 279. Section of an osteoporotic vertebra showing thin sparse trabeculae (H and E x 90)

Fig. 280. Section of a normal vertebra of a young adult showing normal thick trabeculae (H and E x 90)

Fig. 281. "Senile" elastosis of the skin. The abnormal collagen fibres stain black (Hart's modification of Weigert's elastic stain x 90)

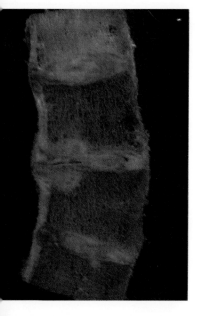
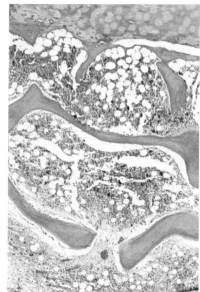
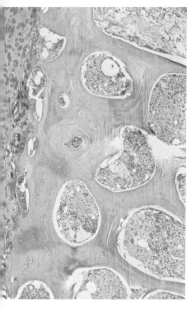
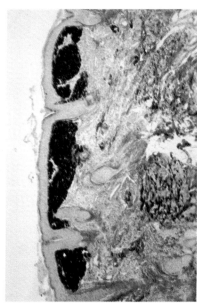

Fig. 282. A radiograph of the upper end of the femur from an old lady. Note the rarefied, porotic bone, a fracture through the neck of the femur and extensive calcification of the femoral artery and its profunda branch.

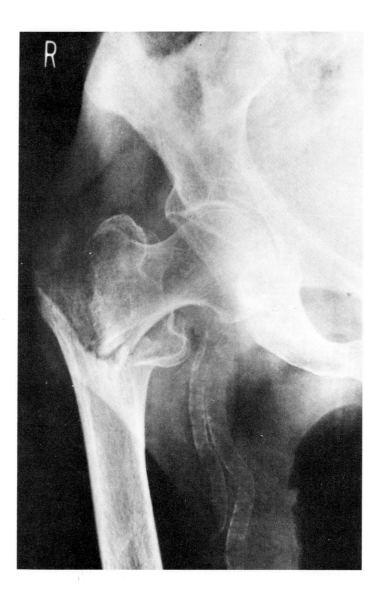

ARTERIOSCLEROSIS

Fig. 283. Blue areas of medial calcification. This appearance is often seen in large arteries of the limbs (H and E x 90)

Fig. 284. Pink layers of intimal fibro-elastic thickening in a renal arcuate artery of an old person (H and E x 220)

Fig. 285. Blue staining layers of intimal fibro-elastic thickening in an interlobular artery of the kidney (McFarlane's modification of Mallory's trichrome x 220)

Fig. 286. Elastic hyperplasia in the intima of an arcuate artery of an old person (Hart's modification of Weigert's elastic stain x 220)

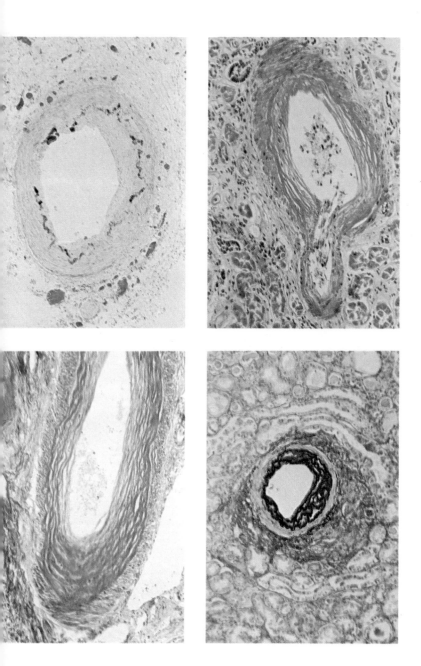

Fig. 287. Atheroma of a subclavian artery showing cholesterol clefts in the intima (*above*), fibrosis of the media below. Only a few elastic fibres (*black*) remain (Hart's modification of Weigert's elastic stain x 90)

Fig. 288. Arterial necrosis in a transplanted kidney. Note the red necrotic arterial wall and the abundant chronic inflammatory cells around it (H and E x 90)

Fig. 289. Necrosis of an artery in acute hypersensitivity (*q.v.*). The lumen contains recent red thrombus (McFarlane's modification of Mallory's trichrome x 90)

Fig. 290. A necrotic artery in hypersensitivity. The internal elastic lamella is still intact though it is often destroyed (Hart's modification of Weigert's elastic stain x 90)

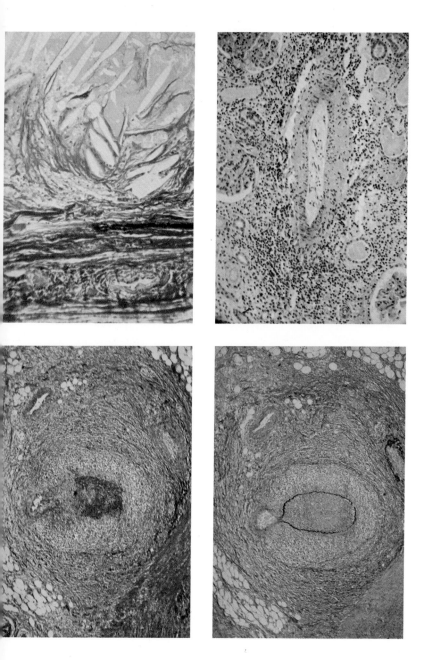

DEGENERATION

Hypertensive Vascular Disease

Hypertensive vascular diseases cause thickening of vessels of all sizes. Arterioles in the kidney, for example, become hyaline, pink and thickened. This is called fatty hyaline change because fat can be shown in the vessel wall. Arterioles in suprarenal, liver, pancreas and other organs are affected and form a useful indication that hypertension existed in life. Intimal fibro-elastic thickening and atherosclerosis are also aggravated by hypertension. All these changes might be regarded as a response to the increased intravascular pressure in hypertension. The left ventricular muscle also responds by hypertrophy of its fibres. This leads to relative ischaemia of the fibres because the growth of capillary supply does not keep pace with fibre thickening. Ultimately left ventricular failure develops.

Sometimes, in the established hypertensive the blood pressure rises further to high levels. No one knows why this happens. When it does many vessels undergo acute necrosis particularly those in the kidney, heart, brain and elsewhere. The appearance is of so-called fibrinoid necrosis; instead of the clear pink appearance of fatty hyaline change the vessels appear smudged blue-pink and necrotic.

Fig. 291. Hypertrophy of cardiac muscle fibres in hypertensive vascular disease (H and E x 220)

Fig. 292. Normal cardiac muscle fibres (H and E x 220)

Fig. 293. Fatty hyaline change in an afferent arteriole and intimal hyperplasia in a larger vessel from a hypertensive patient (H and E x 220)

Fig. 294. Fibrinoid necrosis in afferent and efferent arterioles in malignant hypertension. Note how the necrosis extends into the glomerular tuft (H and E x 220)

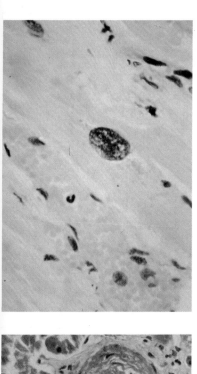
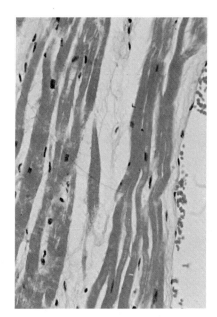
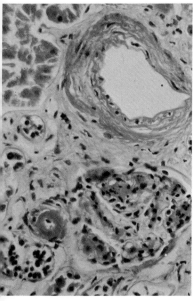
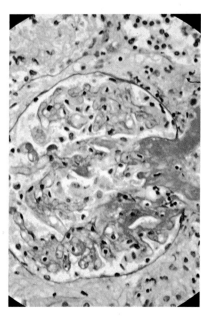

DEGENERATION

Heart Failure and Atherosclerosis

Heart failure may affect both ventricles together or singly. When a ventricle fails it is not longer able to maintain its output so that the reserve volume rises. Left ventricular failure leads to an increased back pressure in pulmonary vessels; plasma and erythrocytes exude into the alveoli (pulmonary oedema). If the pulmonary pressure rises further the right ventricle fails and the systemic venous pressure rises. Oedema then develops in the subcutaneous tissues particularly, of the feet, and fluid collects in the pleural and peritoneal sacs. The liver, spleen, kidney and other organs are engorged with blood the whole syndrome is called congestive cardiac failure. Red blood cells that have leaked into the lung alveoli in left ventricular failure, break down and the haemosiderin is taken up by macrophages in the alveoli (so-called heart failure cells).

Other factors beside hypertension seem to cause athero-sclerosis; those that have been implicated are:

(1) *Dietary fat* and cholesterol;
(2) *Diabetes mellitus;*
(3) *Stress;*
(4) *Smoking,* and several others.

Atherosclerosis seems to occur in stages. In schoolchildren and young adults it takes the form of *fatty streaks and spots.*

These are intimal collections of lipoid with a few cells and fibres. In middle age the lesions get bigger and tend to narrow important arteries such as the coronaries. These bigger lesions contain fat and have a fibrous cap over the intimal aspect. They are called *fibrous,* or *fibro/fatty plaques.* Later still cracks appear in the surface and thrombi form upon them. Extensive involvement of the media with fragmentation of elastic tissue and calcification also occurs in the later stages of atherosclerosis so that the wall of the vessel may bulge out to form an aneurysm. Aneurysms also occur in syphilitic aortitis but the degree of medial elastic damage is usually more severe than in atherosclerosis though it is not always easy to distinguish syphilitic aortitis from severe aortic atherosclerotic disease.

One of the most serious and common complications of athero-sclerosis is thrombosis. This often occurs in the coronary arteries and leads to a cardiac infarct.

Cardiac infarcts often heal by fibrosis forming scars in the left ventricle, most often subendocardial. Occasionally they burst due to autolysis and proteolysis by leucocytic enzymes of the dead tissue. Occasionally after some months the left ventricle may "blow out" at the site of an old infarct to form a cardiac aneurysm.

Fig. 295. Pale staining oedema fluid (filling alveoli) and dilated capillaries in alveolar walls (acute left ventricular failure) (H and E x 90)

Fig. 296. Centrilobular necrosis and congestion in congestive cardiac failure. The histological appearances of the so-called "nutmeg" liver (H and E x 90)

Fig. 297. A central glomerulus has pink amorphous fluid in Bowman's space; this is a feature of heart failure. Note the adjacent blue ischaemic glomerulus (McFarlane's modification of Mallory's trichrome x 90)

Fig. 298. Haemosiderin laden macrophages in the lung. So-called heart failure cells (H and E x 350)

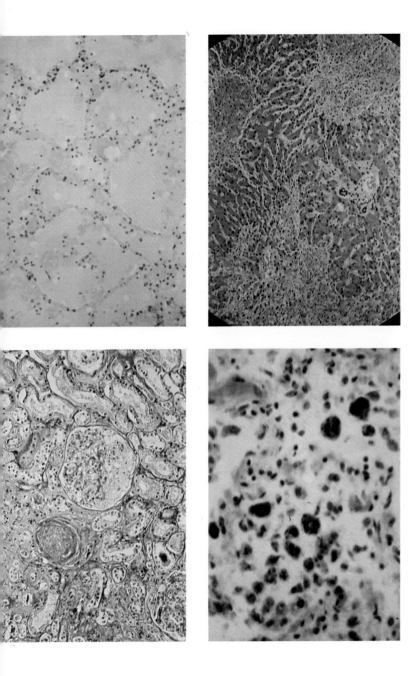

Fig. 299. Haemosiderin laden macrophages in the lung in heart failure (Perls' x 124)

Fig. 300. Coal dust in the lung. This can be readily distinguished from haemosiderin by Perls' method (H and E x 310)

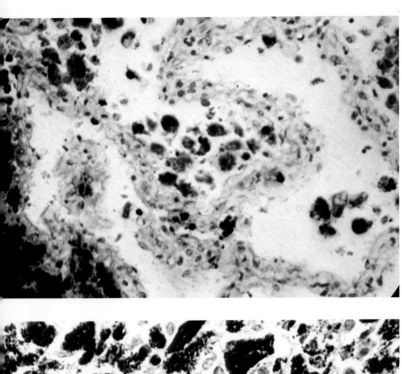

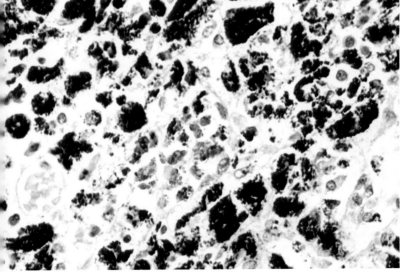

Fig. 301. Extensive fatty streaking of the thoracic aorta in a young man. Apart from the left edge most of the vessel is involved

Fig. 302. An elevated fibrous plaque in the thoracic aorta from a young man

Fig. 303. Extensive abdominal and thoracic aortic atheroma from a hypertensive patient

Fig. 304. Ulcerated, complicated lesions of advanced atherosclerosis in the abdominal aorta

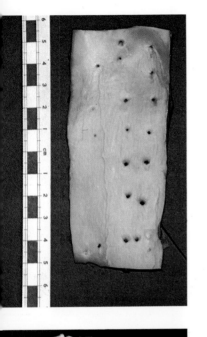
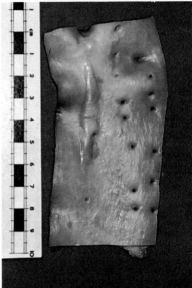
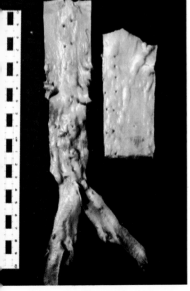
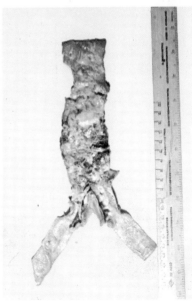

Fig. 305. Numerous, red, lipoid-laden cells in the intima of a fatty streak (Sudan III/IV x 220)

Fig. 306. A fibrous plaque. Most of the intima consists of pink collagen with a few cholesterol crystals in the base of the plaque (Hart's modification of Weigert's elastic stain x 90)

Fig. 307. Cholesterol clefts and calcium (*below*) in an atheromatous lesion (H and E x 90)

Fig. 308. Cholesterol and haemosiderin in an atheroma (Perls' x 90)

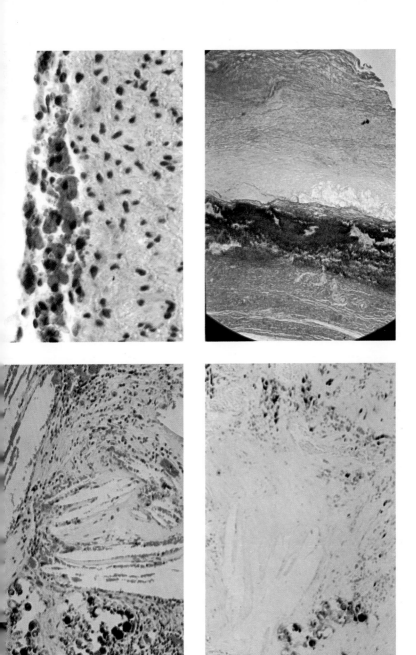

Fig. 309. A few delicate elastic fibres in a fatty streak. Most of this section is normal media (Hart's modification of Weigert's elastic stain x 90)

Fig. 310. A much thicker intima in an atheroma showing abundant cholesterol clefts (Hart's modification of Weigert's elastic stain x 90)

Fig. 311. The edge of a fibrous atherosclerotic plaque (H and E x 90)

Fig. 312. A macroscopic demonstration of haemosiderin in complicated atherosclerosis (Perls')

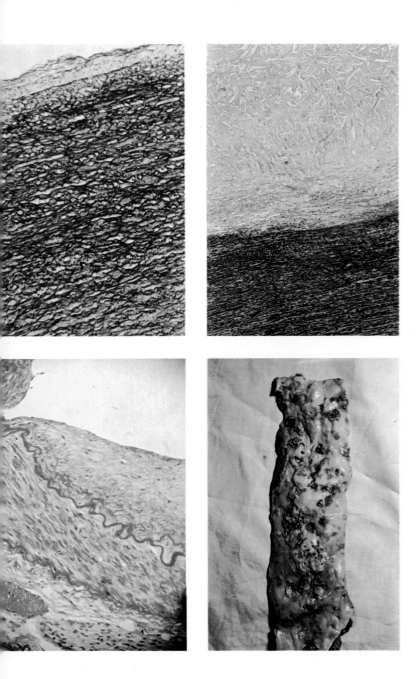

Fig. 313. Areas of medial destruction and accompanying cellular infiltration (*left*). Note the cuffs of lymphocytes in the adventitia (*right*) (H and E x 124)

Fig. 314. Intimal fibrous thickening in syphilitic aortitis. The important distinguishing feature from atherosclerosis is the extensive disruption of the medial elastic tissue (*right*) (Hart's modification of Weigert's elastic stain x 124)

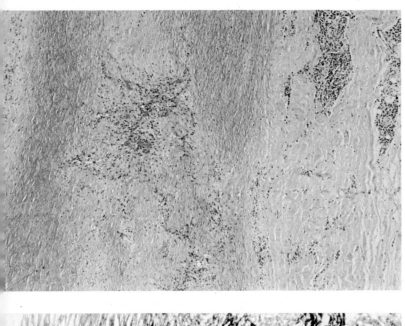

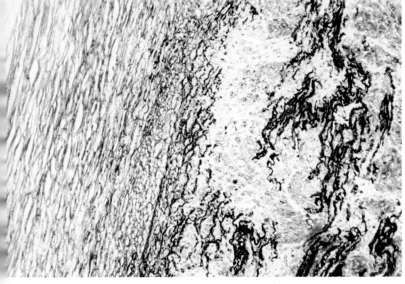

ENDARTERITIS OBLITERANS

Fig. 315. Almost total obliteration of an artery by fibroblastic intimal proliferation. This is often seen in many chronic infections like tuberculosis (H and E x 90)

Fig. 316. Endarteritis obliterans in the wall of a chronic peptic ulcer. Note the abundant elastic fibres (Hart's modification of Weigert's elastic stain x 90)

Fig. 317. Active chronic inflammation in the wall of a chronically inflamed vermiform appendix. Note the endarteritis obliterans and the abundant chronic inflammatory cells (H and E x 124)

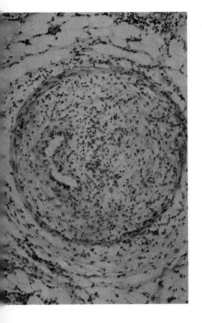
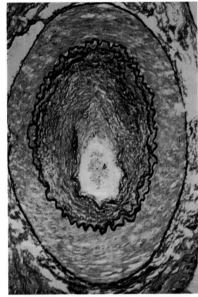
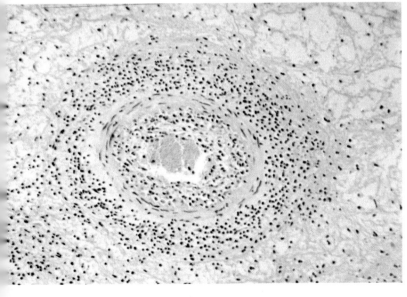

DEGENERATION

Atherosclerosis

Atherosclerosis is a disease of man. It is found in other animals particularly primates, birds and pigs but, in these creatures, it is a mild, insignificant disease usually taking the form of fatty streaks. In man it provides a major cause of death by blocking coronary and other arteries.

Atherosclerosis has been produced experimentally in a wide range of animals by a variety of methods:

Feeding fat and cholesterol;

Arterial injury by scraping, freezing or burning;

Injection of blood clots into arteries;

Feeding Vitamin D_3 and so on.

Any agent that causes arterial damage will produce atherosclerosis. Atherosclerosis can be regarded as the basic response of the injured arterial intima.

Fig. 318. An atherosclerotic plaque in the rat aorta produced by feeding peanut oil. Note the birefringent lipoid (Sudan III/IV polarised light x 350)

Fig. 319. Atherosclerosis in a baboon coronary artery produced by feeding egg yolk (H and E x 90)

Fig. 320. A high power view of an atherosclerotic plaque in a baboon. Most of the cells are smooth muscle cells (H and E x 350)

Fig. 321. Arrow-shaped atherosclerotic lesions in the rabbit aorta produced by feeding cholesterol (Sudan III/IV)

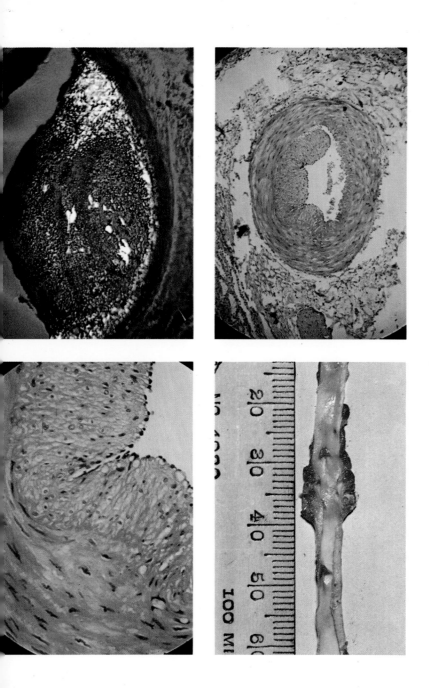

Fig. 322. Atherosclerosis in the rabbit showing clusters of lipoid-laden macrophages on the intimal surface. The rabbit is a valuable model for the study of lipoid accumulation in arteries (H and E x 90)

Fig. 323. Atherosclerotic fatty streak in a pig fed on butter fat (H and E x 220)

Fig. 324. Atherosclerosis in a baboon fed on Vitamin D₃ (100 I.U. a day) (H and E x 90)

Fig. 325. Atherosclerosis induced by Vitamin D₃. There is much more medial scarring than in most kind of experimental atherosclerosis (Hart's modification of Weigert's elastic stain x 90)

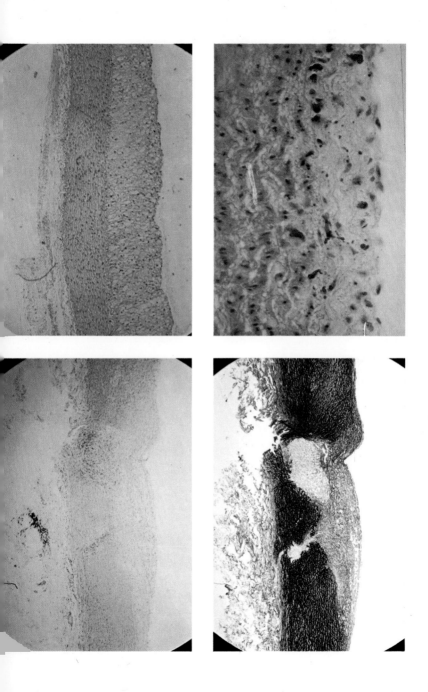

Fig. 326. Fatty streak in a baboon produced by weekly injections of bovine serum albumin. The basis of this lesion seems to be a hypersensitivity reaction (Sudan III/IV x 90)

Fig. 327. Medial calcification in a pig. This is also seen in rabbits, rats and cattle. It probably bears no relation to atherosclerosis (von Kóssa x 90)

Fig. 328. Dissecting aneurysm in the turkey aorta. Note the plaques (*above*) at the edge of the aortic rupture (H and E x 90)

Fig. 329. The plaque is better shown by this stain. It contains abundant elastic fibres (Hart's modification of Weigert's elastic stain x 90)

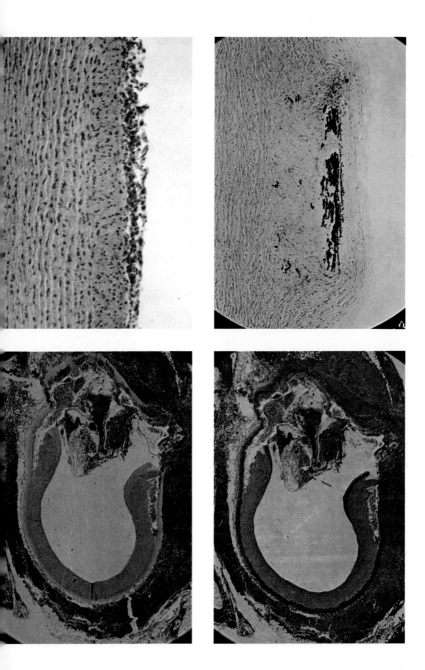

PATTERNS OF DISEASE

Allergy

This word means altered reaction and generally refers to hypersensitivity where an adverse reaction tends to occur when an animal is exposed to a second or subsequent dose of an antigen. There are many examples of hypersensitivity such as asthma, hay fever, eczema, arteritis and so on. Broadly speaking, we can consider four main types of mechanism.

(1) Antibody becomes fixed on to a reactive cell, such as a mast cell, and on further exposure to the antigen an antigen-antibody reaction on the mast cell, causes it to burst and release its granules rich in histamine. This is the basis of anaphylactic shock that may kill; it is seen after repeated antitoxin injections (*e.g.* diphtheria and tetanus antitoxin).

(2) The Arthus reaction which is a rather artificial situation created by repeated injection of an antigen into the same site. After the fourth injection or so an acute swelling develops. This reaction is partly due to the formation of precipitates of antigen-antibody complexes in blood vessels blocking them and causing acute oedema. This, like anaphylaxis, is an acute immediate reaction.

(3) The third type is delayed. It comes on some days or so after a second exposure to an antigen. It is due to the effect of lymphoid cells that carry antibody to the site and react with the antigen when it appears. It is the basis of the tuberculin reaction and of the important reaction concerned with rejection of homografts such as kidneys.

(4) Here antibody is thought to be cytotoxic; when the antibody reacts with the cell surface that bears its antigen the cell dies. This notion underlies the concept of autoallergic diseases where it is supposed that the body makes antibodies against its own cells and this destroys them. Hashimoto's disease of the thyroid is an example where thyroid cells die and disappear and the gland becomes replaced by large lymphoid foci (sometimes called struma lymphomatosa).

Allergic reactions like inflammatory reactions basically consist of the formation of a fluid exudate mingled with cells. A few examples illustrate this point. Eczema is an acute allergic skin reaction; it may follow skin sensitisation by a variety of antigens.

Fig. 330. Mast cells showing that the nucleus is sometimes obscured by the numerous, intracellular granules (Solachrome cyanin x 880)

Fig. 331. Arthus reaction in a rabbit. Note the venule dilated and filled with amorphous antigen-antibody precipitate. Acute inflammatory cells infiltrate the vessel wall and the adjacent tissues (Hart's modification of Weigert's elastic stain x 90)

Fig. 332. Acute dermal arteritis in man; this is often caused by hypersensitivity. Note the diffuse infiltration of the wall by leucocytes many of which are necrotic (H and E x 90)

Fig. 333. A higher power view of dermal arteritis. Note the epidermis (*above*) (H and E x 220)

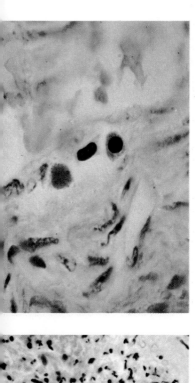
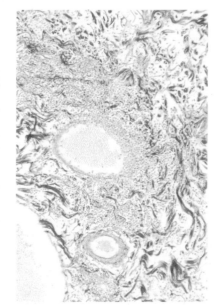
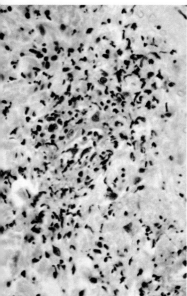
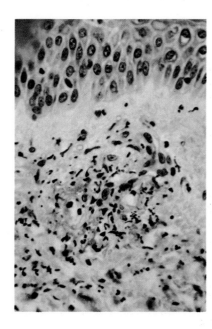

Fig. 334. An early stage of renal homograft rejection showing a few lymphoid cells surrounding atrophic proximal tubules (H and E x 220)

Fig. 335. A later stage of homograft rejection. Lymphoid cells are more numerous; some are plasma cells (H and E x 220)

Fig. 336. A stage of rejection similar to the preceding showing lymoid cells around glomeruli (H and E x 220)

Fig. 337. Many of the cells in homograft reactions are plasma cells (H and E x 660)

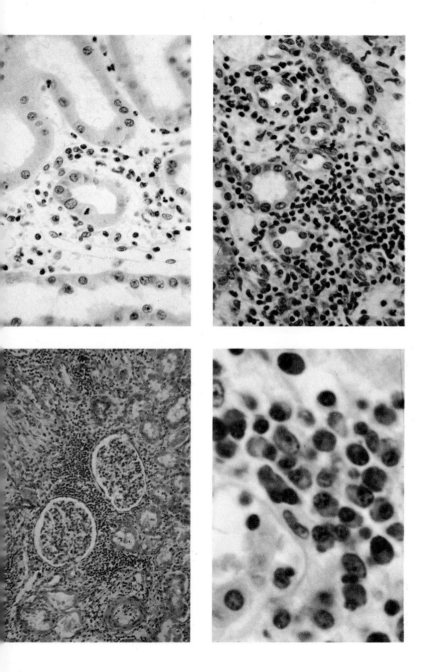

Fig. 338. A special stain shows pyroninophilic material in the cytoplasm of the plasma cells. This is probably RNA and indicates active protein synthesis (Pyronin and methyl green x 550)

Fig. 339. An artery surrounded and infiltrated by lymphoid cells in the homograft reaction. Note arteriolar fibrinoid necrosis (*lower right*) (H and E x 90)

Fig. 340. A higher power view of an artery showing fibrinoid necrosis in homograft rejection (H and E x 220)

Fig. 341. A break in the internal elastic lamella with faintly pink fibrosis of the media in an artery from a homograft rejection (H and E x 220)

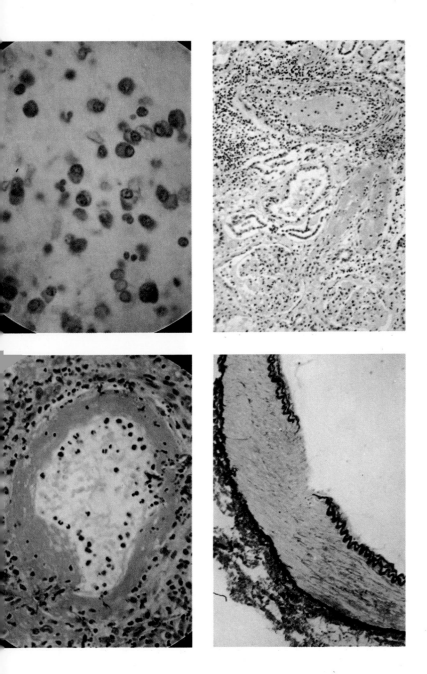

Fig. 342. Almost total obliteration of an artery in the late stages of renal graft reaction. This type of lesion causes a great reduction in renal plasma flow because it is widespread throughout the kidney. The role of deposited platelets as a cause of the lesion is much debated at the present time (H and E x 160)

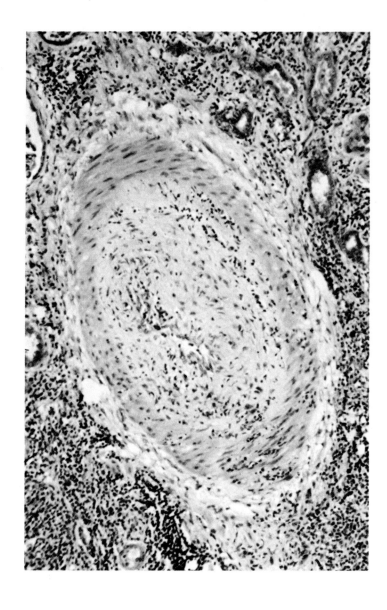

PATTERNS OF DISEASE

Allergy

Asthma is another allergic disorder consisting of bouts of spasm of bronchiolar muscle so that expiration is difficult. Histological examination shows an infiltrate of eosinophil leucocytes in the bronchial mucosa and a thickened, hyaline basement membrane.

An interesting group of hypersensitivity is caused by streptococcal allergy. One of these is rheumatic fever where the joints and more often the heart bear the brunt of the assault. The cardiac tissues swell and contain little granulomas in the early stages (Aschoff bodies). Later this leads to scarring and destruction of heart valves, particularly mitral and aortic, that may become narrowed and incompetent.

Glomerulonephritis is another streptococcal allergy where the response occurs in the glomeruli. They swell up, the capillary lumina become obliterated and many cells of Bowman's capsule proliferate to form "crescents" polymorphonuclear cells collect in the glomeruli. At a later stage this may cause renal failure, though the bulk of cases recover completely.

Sudden or unexpected death in infancy occurs in children aged about three months. They are often male and they tend to die in the spring or fall of the year. The three principal contenders as causes are asphyxia, infection and allergy. The last view is that inhalation of cows milk in a child that has become sensitised to cows milk, may lead to a fatal anaphylactic shock principally affecting the lungs. This is still a largely speculative view.

Fig. 343. Early stages of Hashimoto's disease showing lymphoid cells separating thyroid acini (H and E x 90)

Fig. 344. An Aschoff body in the myocardial interstitial tissue (H and E x 90)

Fig. 345. A high power view of an Aschoff granuloma. Note the degeneration of collagen, macrophages and Aschoff giant cells; these usually contain only a few nuclei (H and E x 220)

Fig. 346. Aortic valve. Fusion, thickening and roughening, with superimposed thrombus in chronic rheumatic endocarditis. Note the atherosclerotic plaque in the aorta above the valve

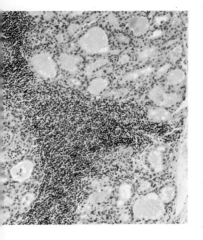
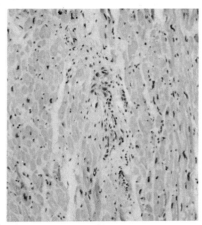
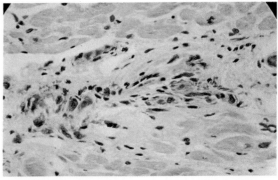
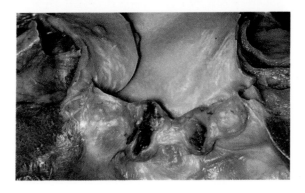

Fig. 347. A view from the left atrium showing the thickened narrowed (stenosed) mitral valve from a case of chronic rheumatic endocarditis. Note thrombi and calcification of the edges of the valve

Fig. 348. Proliferative glomerulonephritis. The glomerulus is compressed by a crescent of proliferated cells. Note hyaline change in the arteriole (H and E x 220)

Fig. 349. Lower part of the epidermis showing intra-epithelial odema (spongiosis) in eczema. Note how the exudate stretches the interepithelial bridges. This is the basis of vesicle formation in eczema (H and E x 350)

Fig. 350. A typical "cot death" scene. Note the carry cot, milk bottle and the infant lying on its face

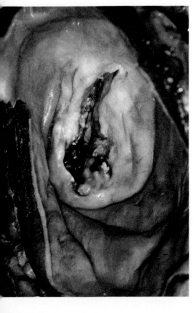

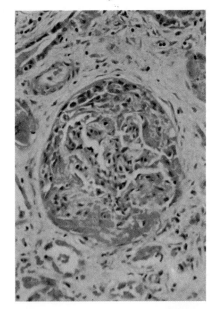

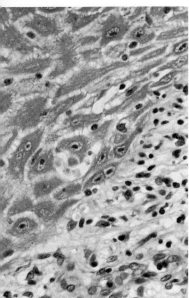

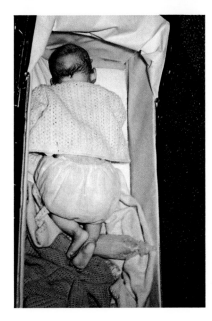

PATTERNS OF DISEASE

Intoxication

Toxic substances are abundant in the human environment, and the widespread use of all sorts of drugs in medical practice makes poisoning a common event.

Carbon monoxide in coal gas and in fumes of incomplete combustion wrecks haemoglobin as an oxygen carrier by forming carboxyhaemoglobin. The tissues of persons who have died suicidally or accidentally from carbon monoxide poisoning are coloured bright cherry pink.

Coal gas was often used to commit suicide. Now that it is being replaced by other forms of natural gas the barbiturates and tranquillisers are becoming more common suicidal agents. An interesting feature of barbiturate and indeed of other poisons is the tendency to cause skin to blister, so-called toxic epidermal necrolysis. The basis of this fascinating reaction is not known.

Many drugs affect the liver, some destroy liver cells (halo-genated hydrocarbons), some destroy bile ducts or lead to the formation of obstructive plugs of bile pigment in canaliculi (chlorpromazine).

Alkaloids from plants of the genus Senecio and Crotalaria that are found in bush tea, drunk by Jamacian natives, have a primary effect on hepatic veins. They lead to a fibrous intimal proliferation that may ultimately block the vessel (veno-occlusive disease of the liver).

Fig. 351. A slice of liver (*above*) from a case of carbon monoxide poisoning. Compare the bright cherry-red colour with the normal liver below

Fig. 352. Toxic epidermal necrolysis in barbiturate poisoning. Note the necrotic epidermis (*above*) overlying amorphous purple material in the blister (H and E x 90)

Fig. 353. Alcoholic fatty change in liver cells; haemosiderin is often present as well (Perls' x 350)

Fig. 354. Hepatic vein showing intimal fibrous thickening in veno-occlusive disease (Hart's modification of Weigert's elastic stain)

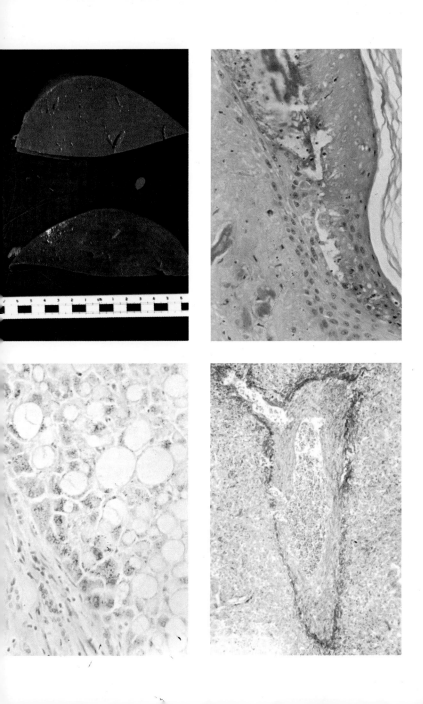

PATTERNS OF DISEASE

Intoxication

Aflatoxin, a product of the fungus *Aspergillus flavus*, has an interesting dual role causing necrosis of the liver in some animals (bird) and neoplasms of the liver in others (rat and trout). The whole field of fungal toxins is developing rapidly; a subject known as mycotoxicosis.

Industrial poisons form an enormous subject and the dust diseases (pneumoconioses) are one small part. Asbestos particles, about 15 um long, cause diffuse intra-alveolar fibrosis when inhaled into the lung. These particles become coated with haemosiderin and give a Perls' reaction. However, not all such ferrugineous bodies contain asbestos and hence they cannot be regarded as a reliable index of asbestos inhalation in life. Asbestos also has a neoplastic promoting property causing neoplasms of the serous membranes (pleura and peritoneum) called mesotheliomas and it is implicated as a cause of bronchial carcinoma (*q.v.*).

Silicon dioxide (silica) causes focal fibrous nodules that impinge on bronchioles and by narrowing and roughening them encourage infection particularly with the *Myco. tuberculosis.*

Fig. 355. *Aspergillus flavus* growing on a peanut. Animal foods made from such nuts may produce hepatic necrosis (x 7)

Fig. 356. A conidiophore of *A. flavus* showing RNA (red) and DNA (green) in the spores (Acridine orange; fluorescence microscopy x 220)

Fig. 357. Hyaline membranes in alveoli .These can occur from the inhalation of many irritant dusts and gases (H and E x 90)

Fig. 358. Asbestos body in the lung (H and E x 350)

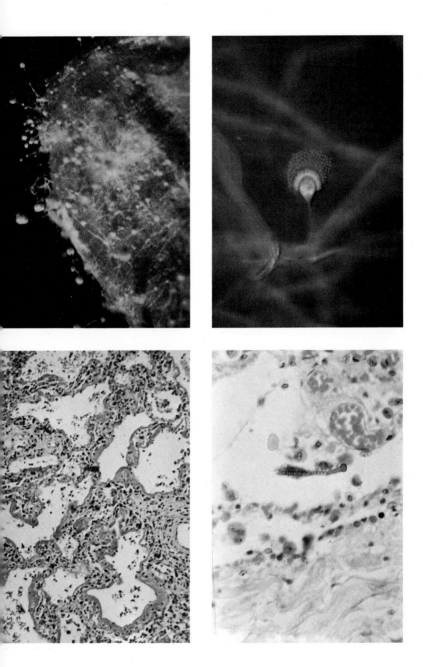

PATTERNS OF DISEASE
Nutritional Disorder

The world is a motley of strange contrasts. In the Western World obesity and all its attendant ills, (hypertension, arthritis, lung infection, gall stones and so on) are the predominant disorders. In other places such as India and parts of Africa under-nutrition is a frequent event. The effects of this are most vivid in the child where nutritional needs are high. Nutritional deficiency is particularly reflected in rapidly growing and actively metabolic structures like bone and liver.

Bone grows in length by the apposition of new bone, formed in cartilage at the epiphyseal plate. Lack of Vitamin D prevents calcium absorption and deposition so that the epiphyseal plate grows as a knob of cartilage that can be cut with a knife because it has not turned into bone. In less actively growing parts of the skeleton where there is mature lamellar bone, rickets is indicated by osteoid seams. This is uncalcified bone matrix and is best seen in undecalcified sections of bone. Calcified bone forms a blue dye-lake with haematoxylin; osteoid does not. This condition is called osteomalacia (literally bone decay) and is seen in a wide variety of conditions where there is inadequate calcium for proper bone formation.

The epiphyseal plate in rickets is swollen. Rib epiphyses form a series of palpable nodules called a rickety rosary. Similar swellings occur in Vitamin C deficiency. Here the basic defect is the maturation of collagen so that the epiphyseal plate is replaced by fibroblasts mingled with blood and fibrin derived from capillaries that have been rendered unduly permeable by Vitamin C lack.

Vitamin A deficiency in addition to causing defective formation of epithelia (cornea and skin) leads, in some animals, to new bone formation. This in the skull causes compression of cranial nerves at their emergence from foramina. Lack of Vitamin B_1, causes defective myelin formation and fatty change in heart and other organs by affecting intermediary metabolism.

Other deficiencies such as a lack of dietary methionine from meat causes fatty change. This is partly responsible for hepatic fatty change and ultimate necrosis in Kwashiorkor, so-called malignant malnutrition because at least half of the children that suffer with it die. It occurs at about one year of age when the child is weaned to a poor quality carbohydrate diet. No doubt vitamin deficiencies and parasitic infections make matters worse in these African children but the prime disorder is protein lack. Carcinoma of the liver (*q.v.*) is a common disease in Africa because it often arises in a cirrhotic liver that is frequently the end result of Kwashiorkor.

Excess may be as bad as deficiency. The widespread practice of consuming vitamin pills and the like may have hidden dangers. Vitamin D_3 for example causes arterial calcification and as much as six times the dose of this vitamin may be taken by regular consumers of certain multiple vitamin capsules.

Fig. 359. Normal optic nerve (*below*) showing blue myelin (Methasol fast blue x 350)

Fig. 360. Demyelination of the optic nerve in Vitamin B1 deficiency (Methasol fast blue x 350)

Fig. 361. Normal epiphyseal plate showing cartilage columns (*above*) and ossification (*below*) (H and E x 90)

Fig. 362. Abnormal pieces of cartilage (blue) amongst the calcifying columns of the epiphyseal plate (rickets) (H and E x 90)

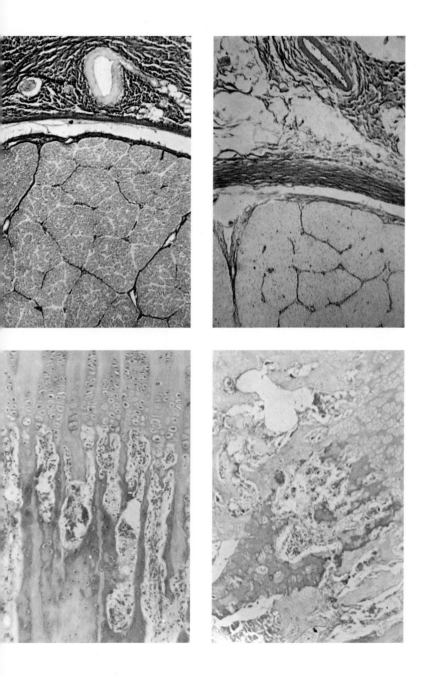

Fig. 363. A pink, osteoid seam (*left*) with osteoblasts on the surface. From a patient with osteomalacia (H and E x 350)

Fig. 364. Haemorrhage on the diaphyseal side of the epiphyseal plate in scurvy (H and E x 220)

Fig. 365. Medial calcification in an artery (*left*) of a rat fed on Vitamin D$_3$ (H and E x 124)

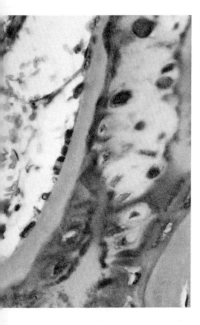
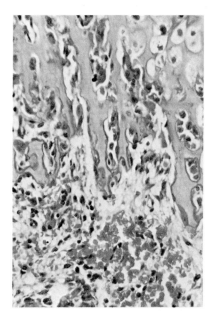
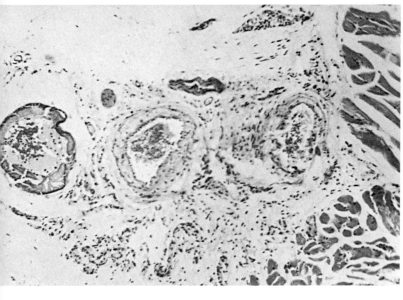

PATTERNS OF DISEASE

Neoplasia

This is one of the commonest causes of death in man. It is an uncontrolled proliferation of cells that is independent of the needs of the animal. The neoplasm may remain confined to its place of origin, when it is said to be benign, or may infiltrate the adjacent tissues and spread to distant parts of the body (metastasis), when it is said to be malignant.

The placenta is a good example of a malignant neoplasm except that it is controlled. It grows, infiltrates the uterine wall and pieces of trophoblast may metastasize to the lungs. After delivery, however, all trophoblastic tissue is shed or disappears; not so with malignant neoplasms.

Benign and malignant neoplasms can be recognized both macroscopically and microscopically. The benign neoplasms have a well formed capsule, they closely resemble the parent tissue in appearance (well differentiated) and show little evidence of cell division (few mitoses); there is no sign that the neoplasm is spreading into the adjacent tissue.

Malignant tumours often have no capsule, are often poorly differentiated and can be seen to spread either into the adjacent connective tissue or along lymphatics and veins near to the neoplasm. Rapid cell division is indicated by abundant mitoses many of which have abnormal spindles and chromosome numbers. In addition nuclei are hyperchromatic; they stain deeply with haematoxylin indicating abundant chromatin.

Fig. 366. Normal placental bed showing darkly staining syncytiotrophoblast infiltrating into the myometrium (H and E x 220)

Fig. 367. A benign tumour of breast (fibroadenoma *q.v.*). Note the epithelial columns in a pale background (H and E x 90)

Fig. 368. Fibromyoma (*q.v.*) of the uterus showing sheaves of neoplastic cells (*above*) bordered by a fibrous capsule (*below*) that contains a compressed artery (H and E x 90)

Fig. 369. Note the red fibrous capsule (*above*) of the fibromyoma. The compressed vessel stains yellow. The neoplasm is composed of fibroblasts (pink) and muscle fibres (yellow) (Hart's modification of Weigert's elastic stain x 90)

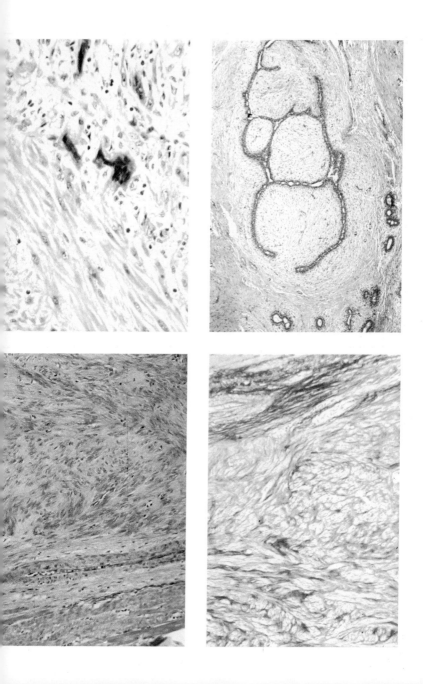

Fig. 370. Hyaline, degenerative change in a fibromyoma. These changes are commonly seen in many benign mesodermal neoplasms and may lead to cyst formation (H and E x 90)

Fig. 371. Abnormal mitoses in an anaplastic carcinoma (H and E x 350)

Fig. 372. Hyperchromatic nuclei and mitoses in islands of an epidermoid carcinoma of the cervix (H and E x 350)

Fig. 373. Loosely separated cells of a malignant neoplasm (melanoma). This lack of cellular cohesion may explain metastasis (H and E x 350)

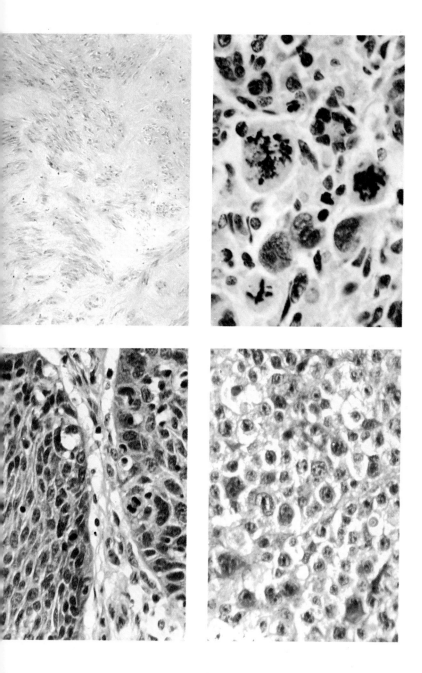

PATTERNS OF DISEASE
Neoplasia (Classification)

Neoplasms can broadly be subdivided into :—
(1) Epithelial ;
(2) Mesodermal ;
(3) Mixed.
Benign and malignant epithelial neoplasms are common. Benign solid epithelial neoplasms are called *adenomas.* When benign epithelial neoplasms project onto a surface they are called polyps ; this is a non-specific term for any pathological projection whether neoplastic or not. More accurately one should speak of an adenomatous polyp or, if the surface is not smooth but thrown into finger-like processes it is called a *papilloma.* Such polyps are common in the large intestine and on the skin and cervix uteri.

Malignant epithelial neoplasms are called *carcinoma.* These are common in bronchus, uterus, breast, large bowel, stomach and skin. They are further specified by prefixing the kind of epithelium from which they arise : squamous celled carcinoma of skin, columnar celled carcinoma of colon. Because the degree of differentiation to some extent determines prognosis this is also indicated in a histological report.

The degree of orderliness is also important ; by this we mean that all the neoplastic islands are behaving or not behaving in the same way. For example, a well differentiated squamous celled carcinoma of the skin is orderly if all the islands produce keratin. If keratin production and differentiation varies from island to island then the neoplasm is said to be disorderly.

Grading a carcinoma is an attempt to define the prognosis from the histological appearances. Factors that are taken into account in grading vary with the observer and the type of neoplasm that is being studied. They are :—
(1) *Differentiation ;*
(2) *Orderliness ;*
(3) *Numbers and type of mitoses ;*
(4) *Evidence of invasion or not ;*
(5) *Degree of host response.*
The host response varies a great deal, generally it consists of mononuclear cells such as lymphoid cells, plasma cells and macrophages. Occasionally other leucocytes are found such as eosinophil and neutrophil polymorphonuclear cells. Mast cells sometimes abound in and around neoplasms ; their significance is obscure.

Fig. 374. Columns of carcinoma cells (*above*) in the breast invading dense fibrous tissue (*below*) (H and E x 220)

Fig. 375. Pericanalicular fibroadenoma of the breast. Note the cellular fibrous stroma surrounding the epithelial lined spaces (Hence the name pericanalicular) (H and E x 90)

Fig. 376. Encapsulated intracanalicular fibroadenoma. It is so-called because the fibrous stroma grows into and compresses the glandular spaces forming long strands made of a double layer of cells separated by a narrow cleft (H and E x 90)

Fig. 377. Normal colon (*below right*) containing mucosal lymphoid follicles. A benign adenomatous polyp consisting of tubules lined by hyperplastic columnar cells (H and E x 90)

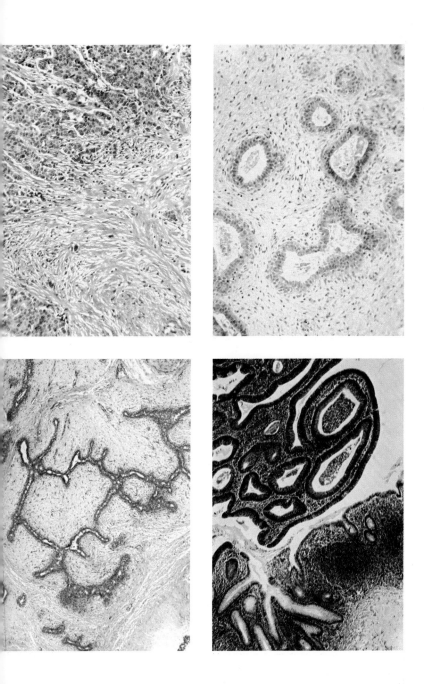

Fig. 378. Several benign, adenomatous colonic polypi. The small one (*centre*) forms a typical finger-like projection (H and E x 90)

Fig. 379. Squamous papilloma of skin composed of finger-like processes of hyperplastic epidermis covered by thick layers of keratin (H and E x 90)

Fig. 380. A transverse section across a benign squamous papilloma of skin showing connective tissue between papillae. Bright red cores of keratin form the surface layer (H and E x 90)

Fig. 381. A disorderly, moderately well differentiated squamous celled carcinoma of skin (*below*). Note that some of the invading islands of neoplasm in the dermis are keratinised (so-called epithelial pearls) (H and E x 90)

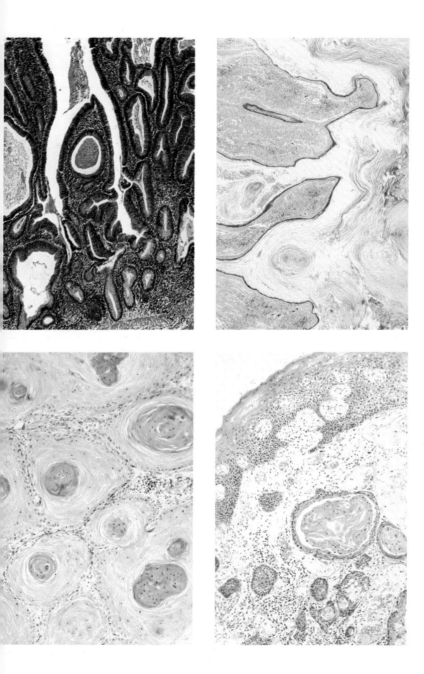

Fig. 382. A duct carcinoma of the breast (so-called comedo carcinoma). Note the resemblance to a mammary duct. The central tissue is necrotic (H and E x 90)

Fig. 383. High power of a comedo carcinoma of the breast. Note shrunken, necrotic cells and mitoses (H and E x 350)

Fig. 384. A lobular carcinoma of the breast invading skeletal muscle of the pectoralis major. Note the resemblance to mammary acini; it is a well differentiated neoplasm (H and E x 90)

Fig. 385. A moderately well differentiated carcinoma of the stomach (*above*); neoplastic tubules have invaded the submucosa (*below*) (H and E x 90)

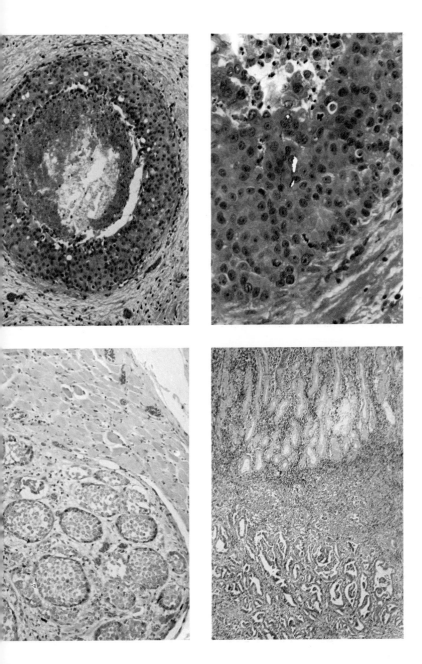

Fig. 386. A benign naevus-celled tumour of skin. This is composed of clusters of melanocytes some of which produce pigment (H and E x 90)

Fig. 387. A high power view of naevus cells (melanocytes); some have produced melanin (brown) (H and E x 220)

Fig. 388. A basal celled carcinoma (rodent ulcer). These are malignant but only locally invasive neoplasms. The neoplastic cells resemble basal cells of the epidermis (H and E x 90)

Fig. 389. Carcinoma *in situ* (Bowen's disease). The carcinoma (*above*) is confined to the epidermal layers and has not invaded the dermis (H and E x 220)

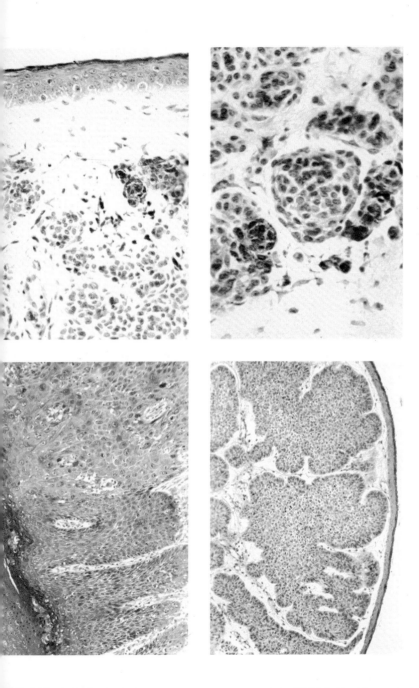

Fig. 390. A dermato-fibroma (*q.v.*) showing whorls of neoplastic spindle cells in the dermis. The overlying epidermis is thickened (H and E x 90)

Fig. 391. A cutaneous haemangioma, so-called birth mark. Note the neoplastic vascular spaces in the dermis (H and E x 90)

CERVIX UTERI

Fig. 392. Carcinoma-*in-situ* of the cervix. A common neoplasm that can readily be detected by the examination of cervical smears that show neoplastic cells (H and E x 500)

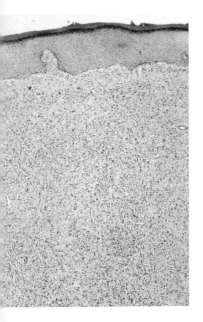
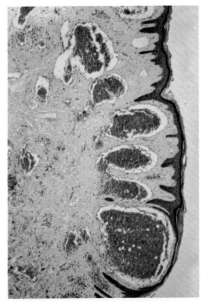
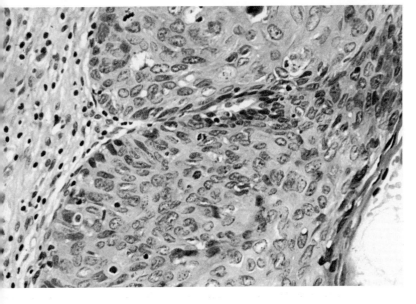

Fig. 393. A collection of lymphoid cells along the border of a mammary carcinoma that is invading fatty tissue (H and E x 90)

Fig. 394. A dense chronic inflammatory reaction (*below*) to invading tubular, columnar celled carcinoma of the colon (H and E x 90)

Fig. 395. Glial cells (*below*) at the edge of a secondary carcinoma of kidney (*above*) in the brain (H and E x 90)

Fig. 396. A cluster of deeply staining, anaplastic carcinoma cells from a bronchus (*below*) in the spleen. Splenic tissue seems to be able to suppress neoplastic proliferation (H and E x 220)

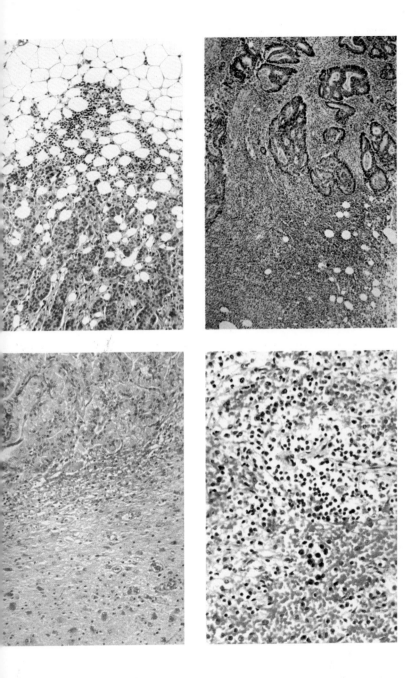

PATTERNS OF DISEASE

Neoplasia (Spread)

Malignant neoplasms may spread in several ways:—
  (1) Along lymphatics by embolism or permeation;
  (2) Along veins and capillaries;
  (3) Along tissue spaces such as fascial planes, pleural and
       peritoneal surfaces;
  (4) By direct continuity into any adjacent structure.
Carcinomas spread by lymphatics to lymph nodes where the
neoplastic cells grow and may replace the node. Some carcinomas
like those of prostate, pancreas and tongue have a tendency to
propagate along perineural lymphatics.

It may however be erroneous to think of the progress of a
malignant neoplasm as occurring in stages starting at its site of
origin and slowly spreading to adjacent structures, to local lymph
nodes and then to distant parts of the body. It is probably more
likely that a neoplasm, from its inception, send showers of cells.
into the vessels that drain it and these are spread over the body.
Resistance mechanisms probably suppress the growth of a large
proportion of these cells particularly in organs like the spleen
where metastases are not uncommon but rarely reach a large size.

Bone is a favourite site for the growth of neoplastic cells from
stomach, bronchus, kidney, thyroid, prostate and breast. Most
bony metastases destroy the bone (osteolytic); some encourage
new bone formation (osteosclerotic metastases).

Lung is a frequent site for metastases particular from sarcomas.
Carcinomas also metastasize to the lung frequently and can
sometimes be seen filling surface lymphatics forming white
worm-like cords on the pleural surface (so-called lymphangitis
carcinomatosa). Liver metastases are frequently seen, as one
might expect, from carcinomas of the alimentary tract (stomach,
pancreas and large intestine).

Neoplasms in other animals are comparatively rare compared
to the incidence in man. Experimentally neoplasms can be
induced by viruses and a variety of chemical agents called
carcinogens.

Fig. 397. Oat-cell carcinoma of the bronchus (*below*) spreading through the bronchial wall (cartilage and mucous glands, *upper left*). This is local infiltration (H and E x 90)

Fig. 398. Carcinoma cells filling a sinusoid of a lymph node. Note the reactive centre (*bottom right*) (H and E x 220)

Fig. 399. Squamous celled carcinoma of the tongue filling perineural lymphatics. Note the nerve (*centre*) and foci of keratinisation in the carcinoma (*bottom right*) (H and E x 90)

Fig. 400. Secondary carcinoma of colon (*above*) invading and compressing liver cells (*below*) (H and E x 90)

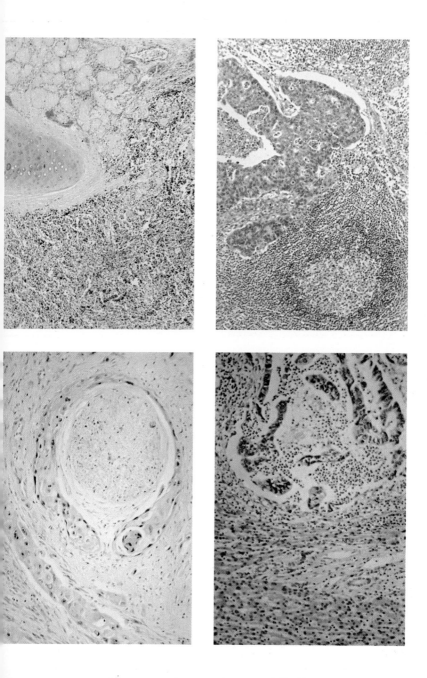

Fig. 401. Oat-celled carcinoma of the bronchus (*below*). Compressed liver tissue (*above*) (H and E x 220)

Fig. 402. Newly formed spicules of bone amongst a malignant neoplasm in the inner aspect of the skull

Fig. 403. White deposits of metastatic carcinoma in a vertebral strip

Fig. 404. Much newly formed bone (red) separated by necrotic islands of a metastatic prostatic carcinoma (H and E x 90)

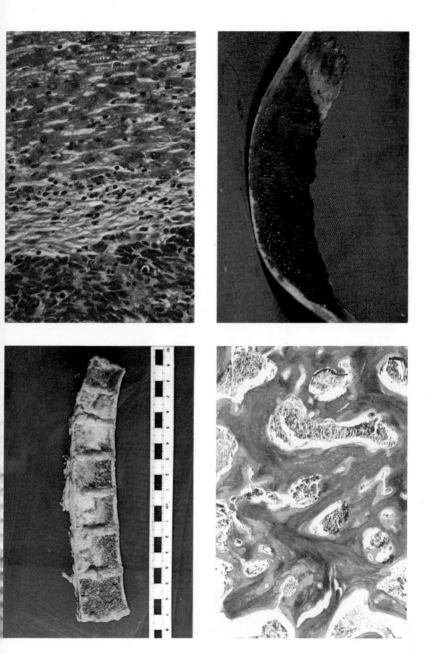

PATTERNS OF DISEASE

Neoplasia (*Mesodermal*)

Mesodermal neoplasms can also be classified as benign and malignant. Benign ones are common, malignant ones are rare. The benign neoplasms have a varied nomenclature which is usually the suffix -oma (tumour) prefixed by the nature of the tissue from which it is derived *e.g.* osteoma, chondroma, lipoma, fibroma. Frequently these neoplasma have more than one mesodermal component in them and hence we have fibromyoma, osteo-chondroma, myolipoma, etc.

Malignant mesodermal neoplasms are called sarcomas. They can arise in any mesodermal tissue but usually arise from bone, cartilage and occasionally from smooth muscle; so-called osteosarcoma, chondrosarcoma, leiomyosarcoma, respectively. Sarcomas differ from carcinomas in that they are richly vascular neoplasms and furthermore the neoplastic cells themselves often form the lining of the vascular spaces. It is not surprising that sarcomas often spread by veins to the lungs.

Fig. 405. Skin fibroma; there is much brown haemosiderin in this tumour due to repeated haemorrhage (H and E x 35)

Fig. 406. Criss-cross pattern of interlacing fibroblast-like cells in a fibroma (H and E x 90)

Fig. 407. Mast cells in a fibromyoma. The significance of such cells, in this location, is obscure (Solochrome cyanin x 220)

Fig. 408. Palisades of nuclei in lobules of a neurilemmoma (H and E x 90)

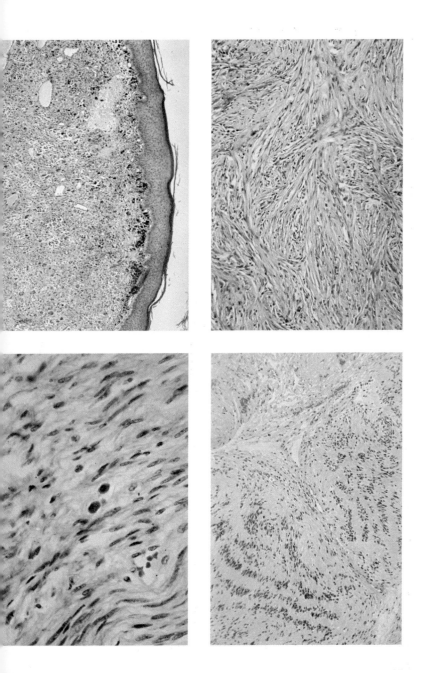

Fig. 409. A lipoma composed of adipose tissue bordered by a fibrous capsule (*top*) (H and E x 90)

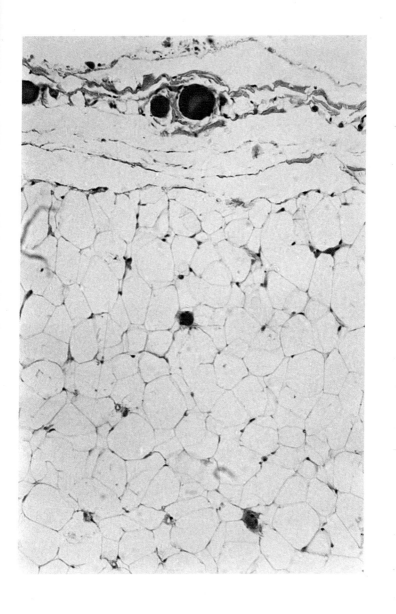

Fig. 410. A group of abnormal cartilage cells in a chondroma (H and E x 220)

Fig. 411. A leiomyosarcoma. Note that the neoplasm is very well differentiated (H and E x 220)

Fig. 412. Faintly pink-staining collagen in a leiomyosarcoma (H and E x 220)

Fig. 413. Mitoses in a leiomyosarcoma (H and E x 350)

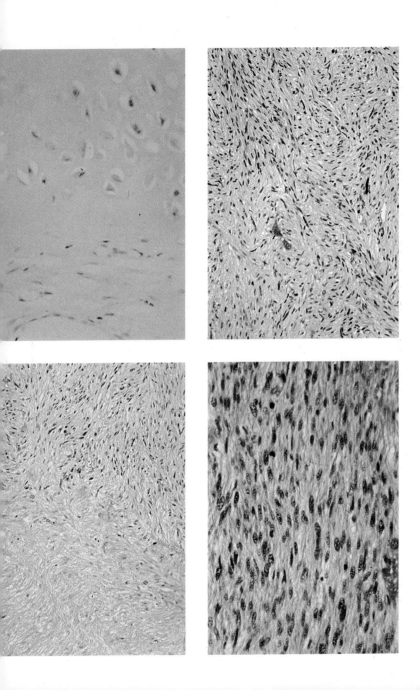

Fig. 414. A chondrosarcoma showing cells that resemble cartilage (*below*) and more cellular parts less well differentiated, (*above*) (H and E x 220)

Fig. 415. A liposarcoma showing the faintly vacuolated cells. Note the pleomorphism (H and E x 350)

Fig. 416. Well defined fatty vacuoles in a liposarcoma (H and E x 350)

Fig. 417. Abundant lipoid in a liposarcoma (Sudan III/IV x 350)

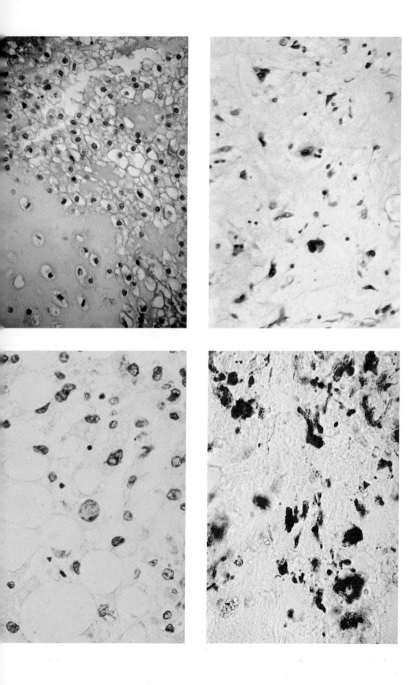

Fig. 418. A benign teratoma showing a central space lined by abnormal hair follicles above, and epidermis overlying sebaceous glands (*below*) (H and E x 35)

Fig. 419. Giant cell response around hairs in a teratoma (H and E x 350)

Fig. 420. Melanin pigment in a teratoma. Choroid and nervous tissue may be found in teratomas (H and E x 90)

Fig. 421. Salivary glands (*bottom left*) sebaceous glands (*top right*) in a teratoma (H and E x 90)

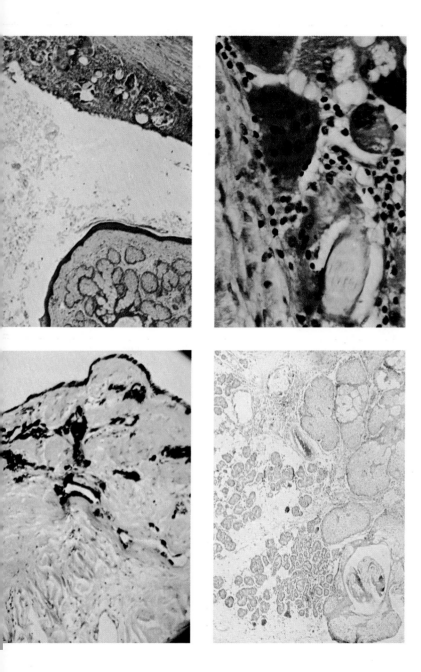

Fig. 422. Lymphoid cells around a portal tract of the liver in chronic lymphatic leukaemia (H and E x 90)

Fig. 423. A high power view of leukaemic cells in a portal tract (H and E x 220)

Fig. 424. Blood film from a case of chronic myeloid leukaemia. Note the abundant myelocytes (Leishman x 880)

Fig. 425. Blood film from a case of chronic lymphatic leukaemia Note the "smudge cell" (*bottom left*) (Leishman x 880)

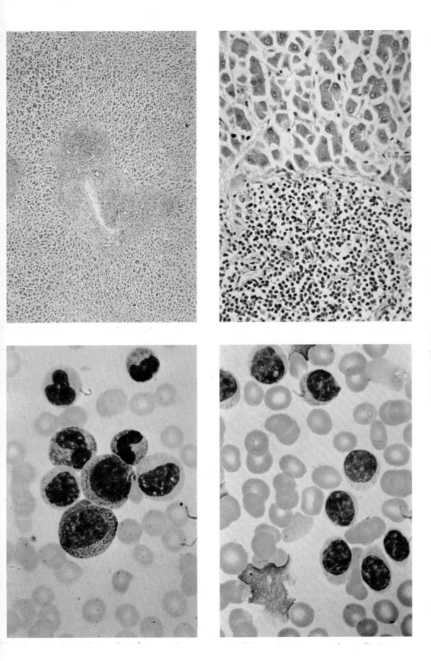

ARTEFACTS

A brief note is necessary about preparation of tissue sections in order to recognise common artefacts that may be mistaken for a pathological process.

Tissue is fixed in a dilute solution of formaldehyde and then dehydrated by passing through increasing concentrations of alcohol. The tissue is then impregnated with and embedded in paraffin wax. The block, so obtained, is forced against the sharp edge of a knife in a microtome and thin sections (about 5 μm) are sliced off the surface. These are floated on hot water, taken up on glass slides and allowed to dry. After removal of the wax by xylene and rehydration in alcohol the sections can be immersed in water and then stained with haematoxylin and eosin. After this the process of dehydration is repeated and the section mounted in a plastic medium (DPX) and covered with a thin cover glass.

Common artefacts are :—

(1) Severe autolysis due to poor fixation of pieces of tissue that are far too thick;

(2) Cutting artefacts due to a blunt knife, a knife that is not rigidly held in the microtome or due to tough tissue such as myometrium;

(3) Floating off artefacts; due to failure of the section to float flat on the hot water;

(4) Staining artefacts due either to improper preparation and use of stains or failure to remove all the wax from the section prior to staining;

(5) Objects of various sorts may become trapped between the section and the cover glass; air bubbles, pollen grains and spores from the air; bits of dust, dirt and cotton fibres, and so on;

(6) Fixatives may lead to pigment deposition on sections *e.g.* formalin pigment and black deposits from mercurial fixatives.

Fig. 426. Creases caused when the section is floated on water (H and E x 35)

Fig. 427. Squamous epithelial cells (*above*) that have been transferred on to the slide from the technician's finger (H and E x 35)

Fig. 428. A crease and crack in a section caused by a blunt microtome knife (H and E x 90)

Fig. 429. An insect that fell on to the section before the cover glass could be applied (H and E x 35)

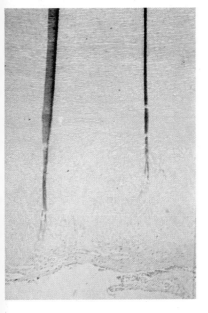

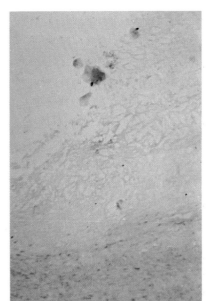

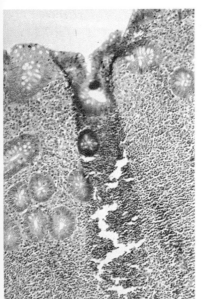

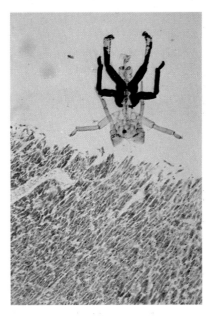

Fig. 430. Creases in a section of liver (H and E x 90)

Fig. 431. Scratches on the section that can be due to a variety of causes (H and E x 35)

Fig. 432. Pollen that has contaminated a section of skin (H and E x 90)

Fig. 433. "Drying back" due to air creeping beneath the cover glass. This is caused by insufficient mountant. Do not mistake this for fungus (H and E x 35)

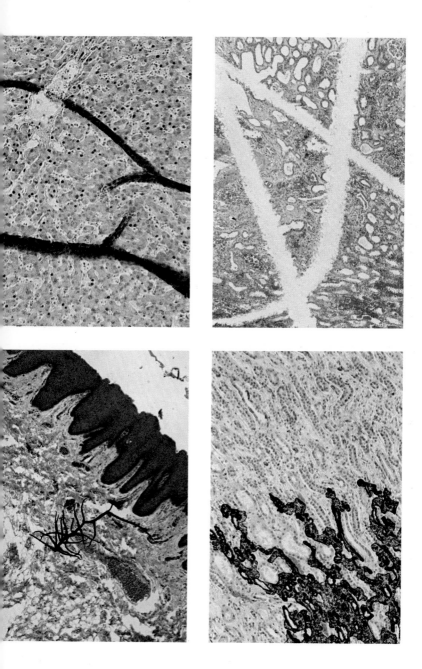

Fig. 434. Brown formalin pigment; a derivative of haemoglobin. It is often seen where there is much blood in a formalin fixed tissue (H and E x 90)

Fig. 435. Black mercury pigment following fixation in solutions containing mercuric chloride (H and E x 90)

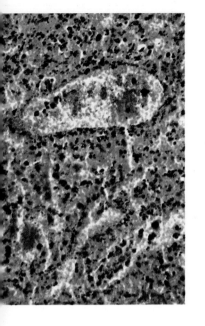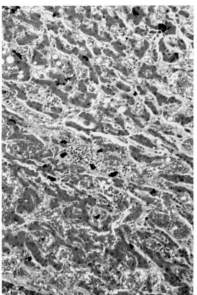

Glossary

THESE TERMS are chosen either because they are not fully explained in the text or because it was felt that further amplification might be helpful.

Abscess: A localised collection of pus surrounded by granulation and often fibrous tissue.

Amyloid: An extracellular deposit of glycoprotein that is deposited in perivascular connective tissues and in basement membranes under certain conditions.

Anaphylaxis: A sudden severe reaction in a hypersensitive creature often associated with histamine release.

Anaplastic: This describes neoplasms that are so poorly differentiated histologically that their site of origin is often uncertain. It may be difficult to decide whether an anaplastic neoplasm is a carcinoma or a sarcoma.

Anisotropic: Able to deflect the plane of polarised light. Most regularly arranged substances, particularly crystals, are able to do this.

Argentaffin: Like argyrophil it means having an affinity for silver salts, but argentaffin structures stain black without treatment with a reducing agent.

Argyrophil: Having an affinity for salts of silver. Argyrophil structures stain black with silver salts after treatment of the tissue with a reducing agent.

Arteriosclerosis: A thickening of arteries. This is a generic term that may be applied to many conditions that lead to thickening of arterial walls. Atherosclerosis is one form of arteriosclerosis.

Arteritis: A general term used to describe inflammation in the arterial wall.

Auto-allergy: A state where the body makes antibodies that are toxic to some of its own cells. Auto-allergic diseases such as Hashimoto's disease are associated with the presence of antibody to thyroid cells in the plasma. Auto-immune is sometimes used to describe such disorders as well.

Autolysis: Self digestion of a cell. Post-mortem autolysis is a common feature of sections from human material.

Bacteraemia: Bacteria in the blood. This can be detected by blood culture but may be a transient effect that produces no outward effect on the patient.

Benign: A term applied to neoplasms that are well defined, well differentiated and that do not spread to distant parts of the body or infiltrate locally.

Birefringent: Synonymous with anisotropic.

Carcinoma: A malignant neoplasm of epithelial origin.

Cirrhosis: This term refers to the tawny brown colour of the affected organ. It is usually applied to a fibrotic liver but has occasionally been applied to a fibrotic lung.

Cytotoxic: This term describes agents that damage and kill cells. Cytotoxic drugs are used to kill neoplastic cells.

Differentiation: A term used to describe the degree of resemblance of a neoplasm to its parent tissue of origin. This term is used to describe the histological appearances.

Exudate: Fluid rich in protein and often containing cells. An inflammatory exudate is an example.

Fatty streak: The early stage of atherosclerosis characterised by intimal thickenings that contain much lipoid both within cells and extracellularly.

Fibrosis: A state where collagenous and elastic fibres are deposited in excess of normal.

Fluorochrome: A dye that renders a tissue component fluorescent in ultra voilet light.

Gaucher's disease: A disorder of lipoid metabolism where abnormally large amounts of kerasin are deposited in various tissues.

Granuloma: A localised, nodular lesion composed of cells that are usually found in chronic inflammations, *e.g.* lymphocytes, macrophages, giant cells and eosinophil leucocytes. Variable degrees of necrosis may be found.

Haemosiderin: A complex of ferric iron and protein that is often derived from the destruction of erythrocytes.

Heart failure cells: Haemosiderin laden macrophages that are found in the alveoli of the lung in cardiac failure.

Hyperchromasia: This means increased colouring. Hyperchromatic nuclei are dark staining because they contain a good deal of chromatin. Nuclear hyperchromasia is often a feature of neoplasms, especially those that are malignant.

Hypoxia: A state of reduced oxygen supply to a tissue, organ or whole animal.

Infarct: An area of necrosis caused by a reduction in blood supply to an organ or tissue.

Ischaemia: A state of reduced oxygenation of tissues. It can be due to depletion of haemoglobin or to vascular obstruction.

Lipochrome: A complex lipoid containing substance that accumulates in cells from aged animals. It is commonly found in heart and liver. Some think that it is derived from the breakdown of mitochondrial membranes.

Lysis: A breaking up of cells. Red cell lysis is accompanied by the liberation of haemoglobin and the cells vanish.

Lysosomes: Cytoplasmic organelles rich is hydrolytic enzymes; their disintegration results in autolysis. Acid phosphatase is one of the enzymes in lysosomes and its histochemical demonstration is a useful means of showing lysosomes.

Macrophage: A large cell capable of phagocytosis. Terms such as histiocyte, monocyte, Kupffer cell, littoral cell describe macrophages in various organs.

Malignant: This describes aggressive neoplasms that infiltrate into adjacent tissues and spread by lymphatics and the blood streams to other organs. They may be poorly differentiated.

Mesenchymal: Appertaining to the mesenchyme which is a general term for the supporting tissues of the body.

Mesodermal: Appertaining to the mesoderm or connecting tissues.

Mesothelium: The cells that cover the serous surfaces such as pleura, pericardium and peritoneum.

Metastasis: The process of spreading of a malignant neoplasm. It often leads to the formation of deposits in organs other than that in which the neoplasm arose. Such deposits are called metastases (singular — metastasis).

Microphages: A term to describe polymorphonuclear phagocytes; usually they are neutrophil cells but eosinophils are also phagocytic.

Microvillus: Delicate cytoplasmic projections seen by electron microscopy on the surfaces of absorbtive cells.

Mucin: A term generally reserved for intracellular mucosubstances as in secretory epithelial cells.

Mucoid: Mucosubstance that is found in connective tissue whereas mucins are intracellular in epithelial cells.

Mucosubstance: A general term to include polysaccharide-containing substances in tissues.

Mycoplasma: A genus of organisms that resemble bacteria but do not elaborate cell walls like bacteria. They have fastidious growth requirements.

Necrolysis: Death of cells accompanied by breakdown of the cells (lysis).

Necrosis: Death of cells or tissues accompanied by visible nuclear and cytoplasmic changes.

Nutmeg liver: A macroscopic term describing the mottled yellow and red appearance of the liver in chronic heart failure.

Opsonin: The name given to serum globulins that promote phagocytosis.

Osteolytic: Characterised by lysis or destruction of bone.

Osteomalacia: Defective calcification of bone as is found in rickets.

Osteoporosis: Deficiency of bony trabeculae. A common feature of elderly women.

Osteosclerotic: Characterised by new bone formation.

Phagocytosis: The property that some cells have of ingesting foreign materials such as carbon, blood pigments, etc.

Pleomorphism: A variation of form. It can be used to describe nuclei or cells. Pleomorphic cells and nuclei are often a feature of anaplastic neoplasm.

Prognosis: This term refers to the probable fate of a sick animal. A good prognosis implies a likely cure and a poor prognosis often suggests death.

Purulent: Associated with the formation of pus. So one speaks of purulent inflammation, purulent bronchitis, etc.

Pus: The necrotic product of bacterial damage. It is composed of dead cells and bacteria.

Pyaemia: A serious condition where fragments of infected material such as pus or thrombus circulate in the blood and block small vessels. Pyaemic emboli lead to abscess formation.

Sarcoma: A malignant neoplasm of mesenchymal origin.

Septicaemia: A situation where bacteria are multiplying in the blood stream, producing generalised symptoms and signs such as fever and shivering and which may lead to death.

Siderosis: The deposition of iron-containing materials in such tissues as lung and liver.

Surfactant: Dipalmitoyl lecithin produced by alveolar-lining cells in the lung. It reduces surface tension and helps to maintain alveolar patency

Teratoma: A neoplasm that contains elements from several tissue components. Ovarian teratomas may contain bone, cartilage, bronchial epithelium and other elements. Teratomas may be benign or malignant.

Thrombosis: A laminated structure found by blood clotting in a damaged vessel through which blood is, initially, flowing.

Torsion: A twisting of a structure. Torsion of the testis for example obliterates the blood supply in the spermatic cord and may cause testicular infarction.

Transudate: Fluid poor in protein such as oedema fluid that collects in the tissue in heart failure.

Ulcer: A break in an epithelial surface. Acute ulcers may heal quickly, chronic ulcers may persist for years. Not all ulcers are infective; some are caused by trauma, irradiation or other factors.

Vascularisation: The development of newly formed blood vessels in tissues. This usually occurs, in pathological states, by the growth of granulation tissue into an area of previous tissue damage.

Vasoactive: This term describes substances that affect the bore of blood vessels either by causing dilatation or constriction.

Chondro-: This prefix means cartilaginous. A chondrosarcoma is a malignant neoplasm derived from cartilage.

Hyper-: This prefix means "more"; hypertrophy means "more substance" and refers to an enlargement of a structure such as a cell or organ.

Hypo-: This prefix means "less". Hypoplasia is a reduction in size of a cell or organ.

Lipo-: This prefix means fatty. A lipoma is a benign neoplasm of adipose tissue.

Osteo-: This prefix means bony. An osteoma is a benign neoplasm of bone.

-itis: This suffix means inflammation of a structure. Appendicitis is inflammation of the vermiform appendix. Pleuritis is inflammation of the pleura though the term pleurisy is often preferred.

-oid: This suffix means "like" or "of a kind". So we speak of lymphoid cells when we are unable to identify the cell more precisely.

-oma: This suffix means a swelling or tumour. It is often applied to neoplasms, *e.g.* osteoma, lipoma, chondroma, etc. It can be used to describe a bruise or clot of blood, *e.g.* haematoma.

-opathy: This suffix implies disorder. So lymphoadenopathy means a disorder of lymph nodes.

-osis: This suffix implies a condition or property: lymphocytosis, leucocytosis, monocytosis refer to increased numbers of the appropriate cells. Phagocytosis is a property that some cells have of ingesting material.

Further reading

This book is designed to be a useful laboratory manual for students. It is of convenient size for use beside the microscope and there is abundant space for the student to make his own notes. The text is brief and to the point. Further amplification of the material should be made by reference to the following books, many of which have been read by undergraduates in this University. They tell me that these books are readable and useful.

Florey Sir H. (*1962 and 1970*) **General Pathology** 3rd and 4th editions (*Lloyd/Luke, London*).
A useful collection of essays on general pathology. Florey's General Pathology does not aim to be comprehensive, but some chapters are essential reading matter.

McManus J. F. A. (*1966*) **General Pathology** (*Year Book, Medical Publications, Chicago*).
A readable, comprehensive text of general pathology. He keeps a theme of comparative pathology throughout the book that maintains interest. If anything it is rather long but is undoubtedly one of the few books primarily concerned with the subject.

Payling Wright G. (*1958*) **An Introduction to Pathology** 3rd edition (*Longmans, London*).
A small book that contains the core of general pathology. It tends to be largely morphological and very few modern biochemical concepts appear in it. It can still be regarded, however, as containing many of the basic principles.

Perez-Tamao R. (*1961*) **Mechanisms of Disease: An Introduction to Pathology** (*Saunders, Philadelphia*).
This is an excellent text of general pathology; it incorporates modern notions about the basic processes. Unfortunately, the second edition has not yet appeared.

Walter J. B. and Israel M. (*1970*) **General Pathology** (*Churchill, London*).

A systematic text of general pathology written mainly for postgraduate students. It contains a good deal of useful material for the undergraduate.

Davis, B. D., Dulbecco R. et al. (*1968*) **Principles of Microbiology and Immunology** (*Harper international edition*).

A useful book that summarises the features of the animate causes of disease.

Holborow E. J. (*1968*) **An ABC of Modern Immunology** (*Lancet Office*).

A short collection of papers about immunology. They summarise most that the undergraduate needs to know about the subject.

Humphrey J. H. and White R. G. (*1964*) **Immunology for Students of Medicine** 2nd edition (*Blackwell, Oxford*).

A more detailed account of immunology. It is easy to read and provides a valuable historical background to the subject.

Waterson A. P. (*1968*) **Introduction to Animal Virology** 2nd edition (*Cambridge University Press*).

A short, modern account of virology. It deals with most aspects of the subject and forms a valuable introduction to the study of viruses.

Disbrey B. D. and Rack J. H. (*1970*) **Histological Laboratory Methods** (*E. and S. Livingstone*).

A short, detailed, comprehensive account of histopathological methods. This is a useful reference book for the student who wishes to know more of the ways in which sections are prepared.

Passmore R. and Robson J. S. (*1970*) **A Companion to Medical Studies Vol. 2.** (*Blackwell Scientific Publications*).

Certain chapters in this book provide a valuable introduction to general pathology. They can profitably be read as an adjunct to this atlas.

Index

Acknowledgements

Mr. L. F. Beard, director of the Department of Medical Photography and his staff provided invaluable technical help and advice in the preparation of this book. Not all the material was made under his supervision and I am grateful to the following for the loan of transparencies: Figs. 23, 268, 288, 334 to 311 Drs. B. M. Herbertson and P. R. Millard; Figs. 359 and 360 Dr. A. R. Jennings; Fig. 112 Dr. P. Whittlestone.

My secretary, Miss J. E. Claydon, M.A.M.S., deciphered the manuscript with great skill and forebearance.

Miss B. D. Disbrey, F.I.M.L.T., and her staff gave invaluable criticism of the pictures and text.

I am grateful to the publishers for the prompt and efficient way in which they have handled the material for this book.

G. Austin Gresham,
January, 1971.